101 'Tails'
of a House Call Veterinarian

DR. FAITH KRAUSMAN

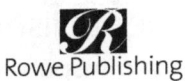

Copyright © 2016 by Faith Krausman
All rights reserved.

ISBN 13: 978-1-939054-65-4
ISBN 10: 1-939054-65-6

Edited by Mary Ann Steinle.

No portion of this work may be used or reproduced in any manner whatsoever without written permission from the Author, except in the case of brief quotations embodied in articles and reviews.

This is a work of nonfiction, however, to protect the privacy of those involved, names, locations, and/or dates have been changed, and composite characters were created when necessary.

Statements and opinions expressed by the author are not necessarily those of the publisher and its affiliates. Neither shall be liable for erroneous information.

3 5 7 9 8 6 4 2

Printed in the United States of America
Published by

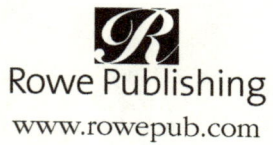

Rowe Publishing
www.rowepub.com

Dedicated to my husband Ron and my daughter Rachel, my two most favorite people in the world, and the reason I exist; and to my mother, Jeanne Krausman, who let me keep 12 hamster cages in my room when I was 10; and to my father, Bernard Krausman, who introduced me to the love of a dog; and to my sister, Ruth Krausman, for putting up with it all; and to Judy Summers, my kidney donor and the one who made it possible for me to keep doing what I love.

Acknowledgments

First I would like to thank Dr. Jay Buchholz for his mentorship during the last two decades. He showed me a thing or two about our chosen field and why we love it.

I would like to acknowledge Samuel Wishner, who brought all of the hamsters, mice, rabbits, and birds into my life.

I would also like to thank all of the clients I have come to know while taking care of their beloved pets.

And I especially want to thank all of the animals featured in this book. Without them, where would I be?

*Strange it is this speechless thing,
Subject to our mastering,
Subject for his life and food
To our gift, and time, and mood;
Timid pensioner of us Powers,
His existence ruled by ours,
Should–by crossing at a breath
Into safe and shielded death,
By the merely taking hence
Of his insignificance
Loom as largened to the sense,
Shape as part, above man's will,
Of the Imperturbable.*

—Excerpted from *Last Words to a Dumb Friend,* by Thomas Hardy

Foreword

Finding a good vet is difficult. Finding a great vet who makes house calls is also difficult. But finding a great vet who makes house calls and whom your animal actually trusts ... wow, that's golden!

Now my cat, Oliver, is very particular. He and I have been together about 15 years, and I gotta tell you, he does not like the box—the litter box—and he is really picky about his food. When he doesn't want to be bothered, he disappears.

What he really, really hates are the vets: their smell, their offices ....

That is, until Dr. Faith came along, and I think because she comes to him, to his house and smells like wellness and feels safe to him, he's all right with her. Now what more could you ask for in somebody who's looking after your animal?

Dr. Faith happens to be one of the smartest women I've met. You will get a feel for who she is when you read her book.

The problem that I am going to tell you about right now will be yours: that is the fact that Dr. Faith probably won't be your vet. But, I can tell you, her vibe rubs off on you when you read the book. You and your pet will be much better off for all of this.

And if you're fortunate enough to have a Dr. Faith in your life, you'll know you're lucky.

—Whoopi Goldberg

Prologue

Why do house calls?

I do house calls because it provides a service that is unique and necessary. Many pets cannot handle the travel or the stress of going to an office. They fear the smells, the sounds, and the sights. They detest being away from home. The cats hate the carrier, the bright lights, and the metal exam table. The dogs hate other dogs and the magnified sounds that seem to be coming from everywhere.

When I come to the house, I see the pet in its natural environment. Even if what I do is slightly stressful, they recover quickly and can be found at the food dish five minutes later. Some of them look forward to my visit.

This creates a nurturing environment for the owners as well. Knowing their pet is in a comfortable space while the exam is going on keeps them happy and calm. They are always grateful and relieved when it is over.

House calls also provide me with an inside look at the animal's habitat. I can see where they are living, what the surrounding area is like, and what their diet is. If I visit a guinea pig housed in a cold basement, I am not surprised to learn that he has been sneezing. If I see a rabbit cage right next to the front door, and it is 10 degrees outside, then I may expect the rabbit to have a respiratory infection. If an owner cannot recall what type of food she feeds her pet, I can just ask her to show it to me.

I can also see how the pet interacts with its environment, with other pets in the house, and with the owners.

These are things that cannot be learned when a pet comes into the clinic, and they provide me with knowledge as to what makes each pet tick. Of course, the veterinary hospital is very important to the optimal health of our pets, but there is a place for both, and they complement each other.

Contents

Acknowledgments v

Foreword vii

Prologue—**Why do house calls?** ix

Chapter One—**Dog Stories** 1
   1. Mrs. C. 1
   2. Can a vaccine be absorbed if the dog swallows the bottle? 2
   3. If you are a vet, beware! Your pet will have a mystery illness. 3
   4. It all started with a guinea pig. 3
   5. The arduous path to the freezer 4
   6. Greyhounds are not real dogs. 7
   7. Frisky 8
   8. The #1 dog 9
   9. Mrs. P. 10
  10. Texas chainsaw massacre 11
  11. This cocker is in control. 11

Chapter Two—**Cat Stories** 14
  12. The Frank Lloyd Wright house 14
  13. Mrs. W. 15
  14. Cargo 16
  15. The marijuana meanie 17
  16. Can animals tell time? 17
  17. Mrs. V. 18
  18. Large house, lame cat 19

19.	Which black cat is that?.	20
20.	My tools are always with me.	20
21.	Feral cats.	21
22.	The #1 cat	23
23.	A visit to Sharon and Ozzie	24
24.	Weird coincidences.	25
25.	Casey, the cranky kitty	26
26.	The Cat Who.	26
27.	Mrs. M.	27
28.	Celebrities	29
29.	Getting lost.	30
30.	The Elvis family reunion	31
31.	Surgeries in the car.	32
32.	No Medicare for cats	33
33.	My scale never lies..	35
34.	Oleo.	36
35.	Cats don't read the book.	37
36.	Help! We're locked in the bathroom!. . .	39
37.	The cat always wins!	40
38.	The cat who could not breathe	41
39.	Mr. C. and Le Pew	42
40.	Don't touch my food dish!	43
41.	Unusual gifts	45
42.	Mr. Scrappy and the nose tumor.	46

Chapter Three—**Rabbits** 47
    43.   Quincy, the rabbit gardener 47
    44.   Poetic justice 48
    45.   Popsy, the bunny 49
    46.   The new bunny 50

Chapter Four—**All Creatures Great…** 52
    47.   Pigs as pets 52
    48.   The "big dog" lover. 53
    49.   Great Danes 55

Chapter Five—...And Small 57
50. Sharing ideas 57
51. Hamster disorders 58
52. The gerbil without a tail 59
53. The guinea pig whisperer 59
54. The neighborhood pet store with the personal touch 60
55. Look in the radiator 62

Chapter Six—Fish and Fowl 63
56. The pond (otherwise known as "Vets can be fish lovers, too.") 63
57. Freedom versus security 65
58. Old habits die hard. 66
59. My organic block 67
60. Teflon toxicity 69

Chapter Seven—Medical Leave 70
61. Life-changing event puts vet practice on hold. 70
62. Will my patients remember me? 71
63. My first day back to work 72
64. Hounds and harriers 73

Chapter Eight—Reptiles and Amphibians . . . 75
65. The iguana lady 75
66. Veeck the leopard gecko 76
67. The mink (or should I say "stink") frog . 77

Chapter Nine—The Early Years 79
68. Get the smelling salts!. 79
69. The farm 80
70. Vet school and music 82
71. Rough start 83
72. Starting the house call practice and becoming official 85

73. Dr. Sammy, the master surgeon 86
74. Veterinary economics 87

Chapter Ten—**Education** 90
75. The effect of illness in pets on the well-being of the elderly 90
76. Light My Way Career Day 92

Chapter Eleven—**The Shelters and the Rescues** 95
77. The dog rescuers 95
78. The shelters 96
79. The rat rescuer 97
80. The bird (and dog) savior 98

Chapter Twelve—**My Pets** 100
81. Lemon 100
82. Herman 101
83. The Syrian hamster, or Shmuel's adventure into the depths of music . . 102
84. Zack, the rat 107
85. Raven 108
86. Patches, the dog with the skin graft . . 109
87. Jaker, the Zum Zum cat 110
88. The dove saga 111
89. Gin and Tonic 113
90. Deputy 114
91. Dumpy, the White's tree frog 117
92. Frogs 118
93. Petey 120
94. Tyrone 123
95. Ricky 124
96. Floyd 126
97. Never bring your 12-year-old daughter with you to a house call at a pet shop unless you are prepared to go home with a new pet.. 127

98. Real or fake? 129
  99. To mix metaphors, why buy the cow
      if the milk is free?. 130
 100. The Senegals or Simon Cowell 131
 101. The longest-living cockatiel 132

Epilogue. 135

Chapter One

Dog Stories

1. Mrs. C.

My oldest client, Mrs. C., was a ball of energy. She was 80 when I first met her, and I took care of her animals until she was a hair less than 100. As a leader of a local rescue organization, she had strong opinions about the community shelter. She criticized them frequently, saying they got everything wrong—from the cage sizes to the care of the animals. She was very intolerant of people who did not share her views. Whenever I would come over, she would have the television blasting Fox News. She was a devotee of conservative television and radio, listening to pundits such as Rush Limbaugh. Her political views were as strong as those on animal welfare.

All of her pets were very old, with dogs older than 15 and cats older than 20. She also lived with a sister, her junior by three years. My technician and I wondered if the house had magical powers, keeping everyone in it alive well beyond the average lifespan.

Mrs. C. had called me to come over to cut her dogs' nails. They had grown too long and were scratching her. At the age of 99, this was dangerous. Mrs. C. had thin skin that could easily crack under a sharp claw. I did the procedure and hoped this would help, but I realized that cutting the nails would not prevent them from scratching the skin. Some time later I learned that Mrs. C. had, indeed, been scratched and had been lying on the floor in a pool of blood. A neighbor had been called, and Mrs. C. had been taken to the hospital for treatment. On the eve of her 100th birthday, she passed away.

Dedicated to caring for animals, Mrs. C. devoted her life—and her death—to them.

2. Can a vaccine be absorbed if the dog swallows the bottle?

I went to a house call for a large dog who needed a wellness checkup, vaccinations, and stool and heartworm testing. We entered the house and went into the kitchen, where we took out the vaccines that were needed. While we were doing this, the dog was very excited, jumping on us and saying a big hello. At one point, one of the vaccination bottles fell onto the floor. Immediately the dog put it into his mouth as if to swallow it. The owner quickly opened the dog's mouth, and out it fell, but I wondered: What if he *had* swallowed it? Would that mean he would receive the vaccination through his stomach? Or would it just pass out the other end unaltered?

I guess I do not have to find that out for now.

3. If you are a vet, beware! Your pet will have a mystery illness.

I work part time at an animal hospital when I am not doing house calls. A coworker has a dog who routinely fills with chest fluid, which he drains and sends to the lab to analyze. The dog has no diagnosis. All of the tests come back normal, including echocardiograms and cytology exams, radiographs, ultrasounds, and blood work. The dog also eats and drinks like there is no tomorrow. Yet, she continues to fill with chest fluid, and no one knows why. She does not act sick, save for a lameness occasionally, which is related to aging.

Many people would not have the resources to do a complete workup on a dog like this. However, we had the referral institutions and consultants at our fingertips. Even with all of their testing and feedback, there was no definitive diagnosis ... because the dog is owned by a vet, of course.

4. It all started with a guinea pig.

I received a call to see a guinea pig with an eye infection. Mrs. G. was a new client, and after examining her pet, I diagnosed a corneal ulcer. The guinea pig was placed on eye medications, and at the recheck the ulcer had healed completely.

After a while, I got another call from Mrs. G. She had just bought a new dog and needed a house call. The latest addition was a beautiful Portuguese water dog, who was sweet and cooperative at the visits, although she always urinated upon seeing me enter the house.

When she became ill from eating garbage, she was taken to the clinic and treated for pancreatitis.

The dog lived a long and happy life until she developed inoperable cancer and had to be euthanized. That was a sad day for all.

A little while later, I got another call from Mrs. G. She had bought another dog, a very active terrier. He had severe separation anxiety and would howl and cry whenever she left the house. With the help of behavioral counseling, the use of a calming diet, and correcting his thyroid deficiency, he began to improve.

Mrs. G was also taking care of her daughter's mini-poodle, since her daughter could not have pets in her apartment building. I had met this little poodle before, at the shelter, where I had done volunteer work. He had come in full of skin lesions as a puppy, and I had diagnosed and treated his condition. However, the skin was never fully normal after that, and his hair coat was sparse. He also had a bit of an attitude as a puppy, and that blossomed into a full-fledged Cujo at times during my visits.

As the years passed, I diagnosed and treated different maladies, but through it all, Mrs. G. kept me posted on how the dogs were doing.

Just to think, it all started with a guinea pig.

5. The arduous path to the freezer

On a cold, snowy, winter day, I had to do a series of house calls on an old dog who was not eating and was weak and dehydrated. He had not been doing well for a long time, and his blood work showed liver disease. I explained to the owner that this was very serious and that the dog needed hospitalization, intravenous fluids, and radiographs. She asked me to place an intravenous catheter at home and start him on fluids. Against my better judgment, I started him on intravenous fluids. He wasn't moving at all, and the owner promised to watch him closely.

I returned the next day, and the dog had become more active but was still very ill. After much deliberation, the owner decided it was time to let him go. Though she was deeply attached to him, she could see he was in a grave condition, and she wanted to end his suffering. I performed the euthanasia, and she asked me to take the body for individual cremation. We transported the dog to my house, where I have a freezer in my shed. My assistant was to bring the remains (which were in a big plastic bag) to the shed while I got the door open and the freezer ready.

A great deal of snow had recently fallen, and my backyard had at least 18 inches of the white stuff, pristine and untouched. As I watched my assistant approach, carrying this 45-pound dog, I saw her pause and sink into the snow. Then, she slowly managed to get back up, trudge a few more steps and sink again. The combination of all of that snow, carrying the dog, and the lack of any path was arduous and challenging. As she grew closer, I couldn't help but laugh as she kept walking and sinking, walking and sinking. I tried to hide my amusement for fear that she wouldn't appreciate it. When she finally arrived, she gently placed the body in the freezer, and we left the necessary paperwork for the crematorium that would pick up later that day. The ashes would be mailed to the owner within the week, in a beautiful urn, accompanied by "The Rainbow Bridge":

*Just this side of heaven is
a place called Rainbow Bridge.*

When an animal dies that has been especially close to someone here, that pet goes to Rainbow Bridge. There are meadows and hills for all of our special friends so they can run and play together. There is plenty of food, water and sunshine, and our friends are warm and comfortable.

All the animals who had been ill and old are restored to health and vigor. Those who were hurt or maimed are made whole and strong again, just as we remember them in our dreams of days and times gone by. The animals are happy and content, except for one small thing; they each miss someone very special to them, who had to be left behind.

They all run and play together, but the day comes when one suddenly stops and looks into the distance. His bright eyes are intent. His eager body quivers. Suddenly he begins to run from the group, flying over the green grass, his legs carrying him faster and faster.

You have been spotted, and when you and your special friend finally meet, you cling together in joyous reunion, never to be parted again. The happy kisses rain upon your face; your hands again caress the beloved head, and you look once more into the trusting eyes of your pet, so long gone from your life but never absent from your heart.

Then you cross Rainbow Bridge together...

—Author unknown
(Source: RainbowBridge.com)

So even though it was a very sad experience, I was relieved to find a small morsel of humor in the path to the freezer.

6. Greyhounds are not real dogs

Greyhounds are sleek, tall, muscular, and sinewy animals. They run fast, and this trait has been exploited for profit. They are usually worked to the bone on the racetrack and then are adopted through greyhound rescue organizations once their racing days are over. They may have been given performance-enhancing drugs that result in health problems later in life.

Greyhound owners are a special breed, just like their pets. I once attended a lecture about greyhound medicine, which was open to enthusiasts of the breed as well. Every car or truck in the parking lot had a bumper sticker stating how much he or she loved his or her greyhound.

The lecturer started off by saying, "There are cats, there are dogs, and then there are greyhounds." He joked that they were a cross between the cat and the dog, putting up a slide of a cat on one end, a dog on the other, and arrows pointing to the center where the greyhound stood. He said, "They don't read the book," as far as lab values, heart rate, or other factors.

Most greyhounds have very high hematocrits, which reflect the percentage of red blood cells in the blood. In other breeds, this would look like dehydration or polycythemia, a condition in which the animal has too many red blood cells, but it is a normal finding in the greyhound. They also have very low thyroid levels, also normal. Many are over-diagnosed with hypothyroidism and treated when they may not have it. Additional blood work needs to be done to confirm whether the dog requires supplementation.

Whenever I see a greyhound, I am acutely aware that its earlier life as a racing dog was rigorous and difficult, with no warm and cozy home in which to live. Many are burned-out from a lifetime of racing. Yet, many are grateful to finally find a rest from that lifestyle and an opportunity to live as a pampered pet.

One such example is Donovan, owned by Mrs. D. He was a sweet old dog with arthritis, dental disease, and a sensitive gastrointestinal tract. He was on many medications for arthritis, including injections of a drug that helped lubricate his joints and rebuild his cartilage.

One day he fell down a flight of stairs, and all of the progress he had made was erased. Though there were no broken bones, he was badly bruised and hobbled slowly from his food dish to his bed. This presented a problem for his owner, who could not lift an 80-pound dog. We increased the frequency of Donovan's injections, and he began to improve during the next few months. Now he is doing well again and is nimble and peppy. But, boy, does he shake like a leaf when I arrive for my visit!

7. Frisky

Mr. H. belonged to Pet Assure, an organization that gave pet owners discounts on veterinary services. Since I am enrolled in the program, I offered 25 percent off on my house calls to Pet Assure members. That is how Mr. H. found me. Mr. H. was not able to travel to the vet easily, so he appreciated my visiting his home.

I came over to find Frisky, a quite overweight black Labrador retriever, who had trouble getting up from a sitting position. I found he had arthritis, skin allergies, an ear infection, and hypothyroidism.

Frisky had a tumor on his foot, and Mr. H. wanted it removed, as it was getting larger and would bleed. I recommended the dog have this done at a veterinary hospital, but Mr. H. requested that I do it in his home—not an ideal place to perform surgery. However, this was a special case.

I gently sedated Frisky, injected a local anesthetic into the foot, and had my technician prepare the site. Illumination in the room was poor, so I used a special light during the procedure. I gowned up, gloved up, removed the mass, and sutured the skin closed. Then I reversed the sedation. Frisky woke up in minutes, with one less tumor and a happy owner.

8. The #1 dog

Randy was a big, beautiful Great Dane with a heart of gold. He was so nervous at the vet office that he would shake and begin to seizure, and became an instant diabetic. The owners, Mr. and Mrs. R., thought that a house call would be the solution to Randy's fear of the office. He was a wonderful dog and a great patient. He had been on a medication for years for arthritis. He needed periodic exams and blood work to make sure the medication was not affecting him adversely. Whenever I visited Randy, he seemed happy to see me, and his blood sugar was always within normal range. Through the years I treated his arthritis, his severe allergies, and a chronic urinary tract infection he developed after being hospitalized for a gastric torsion.

But he no longer shook. Randy was my patient for more than five years. His arthritis was so bad he couldn't climb the stairs, so Mr. and Mrs. R. slept downstairs with him. After he passed away, the owners finally decided they could sleep upstairs in their bedroom. In no time at all, they were expecting a child.

9. Mrs. P.

Mrs. P. had called me to see her elderly female dog named Frank. I knew from the start that Mrs. P. was a great animal lover. Shortly after, she asked me to put Frank to sleep. A few months later I got a call asking me to do a house visit for her two new Jack Russell terriers who came from a rescue organization that specializes in the breed. This is one rescue with no shortage of dogs, as Jack Russells are difficult for many people to raise due to their high energy and frenetic behavior. My boss had a Jack Russell and told me he built an 8-foot fence around his yard to keep the dog from jumping over, but the dog was almost able to get up there. He had a pool in his backyard, and the dog would walk across the cover in the cold weather. He was incorrigible. This may be the same trait that attracted Mrs. P to this breed.

Mrs. P gave her dogs all of their preventive care, took care of their many ailments, including ear infections and dermatitis, and had them microchipped. Their behavior was a challenge for her, but she embraced it. Reginald was always getting into trouble, eating things and biting his owners, while Barbie was a non-stop barker who ate the quilts and began to hallucinate and bark in her sleep.

Eventually Barbie died of liver disease, and Reginald died of complications related to diabetes, but the experiences Mrs. P. had with those two special-needs dogs did not stop her from quickly getting another Jack Russell rescue. She adopted Poppy, who was full of energy and ran away a lot. She was also a barker. Once again the household was complete.

10. Texas chainsaw massacre

We entered the house and immediately had an eerie feeling. It was as if we had gone back in time to the 1890s. The house had been built then and had hardly been updated. The doors and cabinets were a light blue color that seemed very old-fashioned. On top of that, the owners had strange expressions, and my technician suddenly had an ashen color on her face. She looked crestfallen. We did the visit and left the home.

Later, as we were sitting in the car, she explained that to her, the house and the people reminded her of a scene from "The Texas Chainsaw Massacre." She became completely unnerved and was almost shaking.

To me, the house was just a charming old relic, with charming old people and a charming dog.

11. This cocker is in control.

I was checking my messages one day and found one from a woman who was quite concerned about her dog. He had a bad ear infection, an eye infection, and was not walking well. I made an appointment to do a house call for him. When we arrived at the house, two elderly twin sisters, who shared the apartment with their obese, arthritic cocker spaniel named Buster, greeted us. The apartment was covered with religious symbols. The dog took up the entire living room, sitting right in the middle of it like the Buddha, resting on a mat so that if he soiled it, the mess would be absorbed. He was hostile and unyielding when we tried to get him to stand.

We found him to have an oily skin condition, an ear infection with copious discharge, an eye infection causing both eyes to be red and half closed, and he was 40 pounds overweight. A cocker spaniel usually weighs 30 pounds, and he weighed 70. That was why his owners, two frail women with health problems of their own, could not get him to do anything against his will.

They had a veritable drugstore of medications for him and could barely understand what to give him and when. I examined him, treated his eyes and ears, took blood, and reviewed his medications with them. I called the previous vet, who commiserated with me about how hard it was to get through to the owners about the care of the dog. They would be told he was dangerously obese, and they would overfeed him anyway, because he "demanded" it. He was hypothyroid, but their compliance with giving him his thyroid medication was spotty. As for the eyes and ears, he would only occasionally allow them to treat him.

The sisters spent a large portion of their day doting on Buster, "changing his diaper," cleaning him up, and applying baby powder to his skin to prevent bed sores.

I could see how attached they were to him, yet how unaware they were of the harm they were doing. Many times owners are in denial. They think they are making the dog happy by feeding him to his heart's content. Then, when he develops arthritis and various infections from skin folds and becomes irritable and aggressive, they wonder why.

After reinforcing the previous recommendations for this patient, I left, somewhat skeptical about whether they would follow my instructions. The sister who seemed to be the leader, (she was born 12 seconds earlier, after all), ordered the other one to drive to the pharmacy for the medication. Her sibling obeyed willingly, though she seemed confused as to her orders and unsure of the route to the pharmacy.

Even if this dog lived a shorter life due to these medical conditions, and they were killing him with "kindness," he was the master of his castle, and the sisters were his servants.

He liked it that way.

Chapter Two

Cat Stories

12. The Frank Lloyd Wright house

A call came in from a new client. She had just moved to my area from the Midwest and had purchased a home for herself, her husband, and her five cats. I parked the car and entered the house, noticing that it was very unusual in appearance.

It had interesting angles and was very imposing. The rest of the block had average Colonial-styled homes, but one's eyes would spot this house and really notice it. As I entered, I was surprised to find huge, open spaces instead of rooms with doors. The owner told me a student of Frank Lloyd Wright had built it, and they had specifically looked for this type of house.

Unfortunately, there were many high ledges for the cats to jump onto to hide, and the owner had forgotten to place the potential patients in a small room before I arrived. I found that securing each patient was not easy. We examined each cat and gave whatever vaccinations were due, then released them and watched them leap back up onto the nearest ledge.

I asked the owner what she thought the cats felt about this new wide-open layout. She said they loved it. There was lots of room for exploration, jumping, and playing. They had come from a traditional house, and it was like a whole new world had opened without ever having to go outside. They felt as if they were outside even though they weren't.

As I left, I looked back at the house and thought how incongruous-yet-beautiful it was. It reminded me of a book I used to read to my daughter when she was young called "The Big Orange Splot" by Daniel Pinkwater. It was about a bird who dumped orange paint on a house. The owner, Mr. Plumbean, took that "orange splot" and enlarged it to build a colorful home with all of his dreams depicted, even though they did not at all fit in with his block, a "neat street." Mr. Plumbean would say, "My house is me and I am it. My house is where I like to be and it looks like all my dreams."

13. Mrs. W.

Mrs. W. first called me for Paul, a 38-pound cat with chronic constipation. He was morbidly obese and could hardly move. She eventually lost him, and soon after he died, she adopted a cat named Mark, a Maine Coon. Mark would sit outside for hours by the pond in Mrs. W.'s backyard, just watching the fish and staying with Mr. W., who was tending them. Seeing Mrs. W.'s pond inspired me to build one of my own, which I eventually did. Mrs. W. had a poem for every facet of her life. She wrote a book of poetry, and part of the proceeds went to cat shelters.

Mark was very independent and not happy to be examined, so he needed sedation. He later developed diabetes, and Mr. W. faithfully gave him insulin twice a day. If there were any problems, I would come by to examine him. Mrs. W. had declining vision, but she had a keen sense of knowing how Mark was feeling on any given day. When she thought he was "off," she was usually right. Mark had gone through nine lives and passed away at the age of 23, near the pond where he had always loved to sit and watch the fish.

14. Cargo

One day a truck driver brought in a cat to the veterinary hospital where I work part time. The cat had been hiding in a shipment of matzo (unleavened bread that is eaten during the Jewish holiday of Passover) from Israel that he was delivering to a store. As he was unloading the truck, he discovered the stowaway in one of the boxes. How the cat had survived the trip was a mystery, but since the truck driver now felt responsible for his passenger, he brought him in for an exam.

We found mild dehydration, and the cat was very thin. Otherwise, everything appeared to be normal. The cat had never gone through any checks at the airport since he had been "smuggled" in, so I called the airport security to ask them what to do. They requested the animal be quarantined for several weeks and tested for leishmania, a parasitic disease that is not uncommon in its country of origin.

The quarantine went well, we updated his vaccinations, and the trucker adopted him and named him Cargo. He would come in yearly for his exam.

Just recently, the owner had him put to sleep, now an old, sick kitty. But Cargo had an unexpected and beautiful life, thanks to his ingenuity going into that box of matzo.

He might be the first feline illegal alien!

15. The marijuana meanie

My technician and I went to see an elderly woman who had adopted a cat from a shelter and wanted to have her examined. She thought the cat had a skin allergy and an ear infection.

The woman had suffered a stroke and was being treated with medical marijuana, which we could smell as soon as we entered her bedroom. To our surprise, instead of her being mellow from the pot, she was meaner than ever. She kept ordering us to do this or that with the cat, and when we couldn't oblige her, she started yelling.

The cat was on her bed while we examined her, and this made things more stressful for all concerned. I did the best I could to satisfy this client's demands, but there was no pleasing her. We left there slightly disconcerted, imagining how she would have acted if the marijuana had not been on board.

16. Can animals tell time?

Several times I did a house call for an elderly woman who owned a cat. As I entered her house and collected my examination tools, she explained that her cat was her connection to reality. He "told" her when to feed him by sitting near the cabinet containing his food and meowing.

He sat by her feet as she watched television at night, but at a certain time each night he would get up and tell her it was bedtime. Then he would coax her to go upstairs. In the morning, he would nudge her awake, telling her it was time to get up. "I don't know what I would do without him. He keeps me in a routine and is better than a wrist watch," she said.

The owner was getting less mobile as she got older and was losing some of her hearing and vision, so the cat helped her maintain her autonomy and continue with her organized life.

I find this is true for many of us. Our pets keep reminding us what time it is and make us focus on the most basic things in our lives: when to get up, when to eat, when to go out for a walk, when to rest, when to eat again, when to sleep. By doing this, they keep us on a schedule.

Can animals tell time?

Definitely. Not by the minute or the hour, but they do have internal clocks.

17. Mrs. V.

Mrs. V. came to the first hospital at which I worked in New Jersey and followed me to every succeeding practice. She had more than 50 cats and a few dogs. She was also an officer of a volunteer organization that tried to get pets spayed, neutered, and adopted. The motto of the organization was, "Don't breed or buy while homeless pets die."

She loved cats dearly and was always bringing in one or two with an illness. They would usually be emaciated and dehydrated, and, more often than not, were suffering from a chronic disease such as kidney failure or diabetes. Mrs. V. always thought a cat was okay as long as he or she was eating. She had her own ideas about the best cat foods to feed.

While she was in the office she would befriend everyone else in the waiting room. She knew every staff member's name and came to some of our weddings and other celebrations. If she saw us working late at the office, she would come back with a couple of pizzas. She always remembered us at the holidays and would spend her last penny on a sick pet. I never saw Mrs. V. at her house to treat her cats. Perhaps she wanted to avoid having me see the monumental number of cats she had there. I think, for her, the hospital was like a second home. She named a cat after me, which was quite an honor. Mrs. V. was one of a kind.

18. Large house, lame cat

We entered the house and were greeted by the mom, dad, and daughter. The cat had been put in a bathroom, as instructed. Many times a cat will run and hide if allowed to roam throughout the house with a vet in the vicinity. This house was so big that one could get lost just trying to find the way out.

The cat was a 13-year-old indoor/outdoor female who had been taken to another vet when she had started limping. The doctor had taken an X-ray of the leg, found no fracture, and treated symptomatically with anti-inflammatory medication. Instead of improving, she had become increasingly lame. When examining her, I found that she felt a great deal of pain in the hip. When I recommended more diagnostics, the owner told me in no uncertain terms that she was not attached to the cat, so please, no big bills.

This cat was the only surviving cat of a litter of four, the others having met one disaster or another during their outside adventures. Although this cat did go out, she thus far had managed to escape the others' fates.

How does one live with a cat for 13 years and not get attached? She may not have realized it, but she was attached.

19. Which black cat is that?

I have always loved black cats. I had Raven, who lived until age 21, and Floyd, who is 16 and still a mensch. But I did not have them both at the same time.

When I do a house call in a multiple-cat household, I usually see a variety of colors. The cats may range from black to white, to calico, to tortoiseshell, to tiger, to orange, to grey. Recently I went on a house call in which there were five cats, all black. They had come from various sources, such as craigslist, a rescue, the street, or from a person who had to find a new home for his pet. The owners said each one had a special trait—one with a long chin, one with more upright ears, one very thin, one with a small white spot, and one with a paunch. As far as these owners were concerned, each of their cats was an individual, and they looked beyond color.

We should all be so colorblind.

20. My tools are always with me.

Twice I visited a cat to do a physical exam. The first time I forgot to bring my black doctor's bag, and the second time I left the cooler at home. The black bag contains a stethoscope and ophthalmoscope, while the cold bag contains vaccinations and injectable antibiotics.

In both cases, I did fine. I realized I did not need my black bag to do a good exam. I had my eyes for seeing, my ears for hearing, and my hands for palpating. I also did not need anything from my cooler, as I was not administering vaccinations or antibiotics. What this taught me was that I am always carrying my tools, for they are within me, not beyond me. The art of physical diagnosis centers mostly on listening to a patient's history and performing a hands-on, thorough physical exam. We have become too dependent on all of our "outer tools" and have lost touch with our "inner tools." This was a wake-up call to remind me of what I possess. The strange part of this is why only this particular cat? Did she cast a magic spell on me both times to induce memory loss? We'll see what happens on the next visit.

21. Feral cats

To a house call vet, feral cats are always a challenge. These cats sometimes end up indoors as pets but can't be touched and must be admired from a distance. It is an inborn trait to fear humans, so they hide and run as far away from me as possible when I visit. I have one client who is a "Cat Lady" with 12 of them in the house and 15 more outside. She provides food and igloo shelters for them, and they are quite content. About four of her indoor cats are feral, and they are intractable and will never trust humans. That is when she calls me.

I saddle up with sedatives, eat my Wheaties, and sharpen my reflexes for the visit. Once I arrive, Cat Lady directs me to the bathroom, where I quickly open and close the door behind me.

Connie is in the corner of the storage closet, facing the wall. I give her an injection of a sedative, grabbing the towel to shield myself as I reach around to do this, preventing a counter attack. Once completed,

I wait patiently for it to take effect. I stay very quiet, employing yoga poses to unravel my spine from the tension that just built up there. In about 10 minutes, she becomes sedated, and I gently move her from the closet, place her on the towel, and call in my assistant.

I perform a physical exam, take blood, fecal and urine samples, and give her vaccinations. We lubricate her eyes so they don't become dry. I then apply flea preventative. When we are finished, I give her subcutaneous fluids to help her have a smooth recovery. Then we quickly clear out of the bathroom before she wakes up. When she does, she will remember it as only a bad dream. I tell the owner my findings, and as I have done every year, I add the phrase, "This is the last time I come to see Connie! I'm getting too old for this!"

Mr. S. is another owner who caters to feral cats. He has some indoor cats, but he looks after an outdoor colony as well. He brings in a cat to spay or neuter every few months and puts them back into their colony to live out their lives. Except for Twilight, who had started out as an outside cat, a big guy who was very fearsome. Mr. S. trapped him and brought him to be neutered, but there was something about Twilight. He wasn't like the other cats. He had a certain quality, a *je ne sais quoi*. Mr. S. was smitten. He would take him in.

The first clue that something was wrong with Twilight was that he had a fever of 104.8 and had upper airway congestion and severe dental disease. He also had an unkempt hair coat and conjunctivitis. In short, he was a mess. His FeLV/FIV test came up positive for FIV, feline immunodeficiency virus, which is also called feline AIDs. It was first discovered in cats in the 1980s and results in a reduced immune response.

It can lead to severe dental disease, ear infections, subcutaneous abscesses, conjunctivitis, respiratory disease, seizures, kidney disease, and lymphoma, a form of cancer.

Twilight was first treated for infection and kept indoors until he was feeling better. Mr. S. kept him away from his other cats as FIV is contagious and can be transmitted by bite wounds or the exchange of body fluids. Two weeks later, Twilight had his neuter procedure and a dental. From then on, he was on antibiotics intermittently for his chronic respiratory infection. He had radiographs, tracheal washes, blood tests, eye drops, and oral medications, but never really improved. He was treated for pneumonia and asthma and was hospitalized on and off for three years. Every antimicrobial drug was used on this cat. In addition to all of this, he developed large kidneys, large abdominal lymph nodes, a large spleen, and a nodule in the left lung. The diagnosis was lymphoma, an invasive cancer that is common in cats. Twilight passed away, and the following is a sympathy note from my boss:

"It was an honor to care for Twilight over the years, and I can honestly say he was a favorite patient of mine (tough as he was). From the moment he came into your life, you gave him the best chance possible. You gave him a great quality of life and an exceptionally loving home. 'Best friends are never forgotten; they live on in our hearts forever.'"

One can see why people take in feral cats.

22. The #1 cat

Frecka the cat was 20 years old and had kidney disease and hyperthyroidism. Her owner, Mrs. B., was 97, had lost her vision in her 80s, and was hard of hearing. I came by three times a week to give fluids, perform an exam, and occasionally take blood. Every time I came over, Mrs. B. would perk up, so happy I was there. She could never find the door to let me in and would create loud clanging noises until she located it. Frecka enjoyed her treatment and was visibly improving within minutes of getting her fluid injection. When I saw the way both Frecka and her owner became more animated, more content, and more inclined to be social after this treatment, it made me decide to do a study on how illness in pets affects their elderly owners. She was the inspiration for my work on this topic.

I continued treating Frecka for years, until she had too many medical problems to which she eventually succumbed. After that, Mrs. B.'s health declined as well, and she died a short while later, not quite reaching 100.

23. A visit to Sharon and Ozzie

The sign on the door was fastened with tape. It read, "Welcome Pet Lovers. Come In." We were expected at 9 a.m. The door was open, so after knocking gently, we entered. There we saw the cat we needed to examine, sitting on the couch. A bad feeling crept over me. Cats were supposed to be placed in the bathroom before our arrival.

Once I arrive, all bets are off. They smell "DOCTOR" and run for the hills. I asked the owner if she could place Sharon, her 4-year-old, black-and-white cat in the bathroom. To our great fortune, she picked her up, brought her upstairs, and after what sounded like a brief struggle, wrangled her into the bathroom.

Ozzie, the other cat, happily looked on, curious, and satisfied in knowing he wasn't being examined that day. Sharon's exam went smoothly. She had a heart murmur, dental disease, and was overweight. We gave treatment recommendations and said we hoped she didn't get too upset by our visit. Judging by the way she stretched out on the bed shortly after, I would say she was just fine.

Ozzie, we'll be coming back to see you soon.

24. Weird coincidences

Weird coincidences happen in my house call schedule. For example, I visited this one household with four dogs on the same day I visited the owner's mother-in-law's dog. This happened three times.

Another coincidence was that every time I was called to help at the shelter with zeutering (a non-surgical castration technique), I had a certain house call scheduled in a home with four cats. This happened twice.

I recently saw Chatty Kathy, a cat who needed a recheck for a bite wound. She was sore around her tail and had improved on antibiotics. We were going to see her again the following week for her annual visit and vaccinations. On our way to the next visit, we received a call from a new client named Kathy.

My technician was fielding many questions from the caller, such as, "Why do you need a towel to get into the bathroom?" to "Why are your fees higher than the article says on your website?" (The article had been written eight years prior!) My technician finished the call, a bit frustrated. I asked her what time she had scheduled the appointment. It turned out to be right after Chatty Kathy's appointment. "Looks like we have one 'Chatty Kathy' after another that day," I said.

25. Casey, the cranky kitty

When I first met Casey he weighed 26 pounds and was very mellow. As a cat whose ideal weight was 15 pounds, he was considered obese. He was also diabetic and on insulin. As I studied this case, I thought it best to put Casey on an aggressive weight-management plan. We ran a weight loss contest at the office, and Mrs. O., his owner, was eager to participate. I would guess Casey was not so eager, but before you knew it, he had lost a lot of weight, and he won the contest! And his diabetes went into remission.

However, as I continued to visit him at the house, he became less willing to let me handle him. In fact he was less sweet, in more ways than one. He had other health problems, including a large kidney and a history of being blocked, a term used to describe when a cat cannot urinate because the urethra is plugged with crystals, mucus plugs, or both. This can be seasonal, as more cats become blocked when the weather changes. It is linked to stress, diet, and other factors. The treatment is to pass a urinary catheter, flush the obstruction out, and give intravenous fluids and medications. In some cases, surgery (perineal urethrostomy) is required to create a larger opening through which the male cat can urinate. Casey had the PU surgery, which relieved his urinary problem.

Casey had become so anti-social that the only thing he would let us do was a brief exam and a weight. Although he is now svelte and no longer diabetic, he is very bossy and has quite an attitude.

26. The Cat Who

Whenever I visited a certain client (who owned an elderly cat), she would lend me one of "The Cat Who" series by Lillian Jackson Braun. These books were about Jim Qwilleran, an older man who solved crime mysteries with the help of his two Siamese cats, Koko and Yum Yum. He was an expert sleuth—or was it his cats who were the great detectives?

At each visit I would return the last book and receive another. Qwilleran was not only a master detective, but he also loved antiques, and a large part of each book was devoted to that subject.

He always gave his cats clam juice as a treat. I thought how clever that was. Without realizing it, he was protecting them from a very serious heart ailment called feline dilated cardiomyopathy. In this disease, cats develop a flabby heart muscle, which cannot pump efficiently. This leads to congestive heart failure. In the 1980s, a discovery was made that showed that taurine deficiency contributed to this problem. Supplementing the diet with this amino acid resulted in cats not developing this disease. Those who already had the disease would improve. That study led to putting taurine into all cat foods.

Qwilleran knew nothing of this, yet he gave his cats clam juice, a great source of this necessary substance, so they were protected from this disease and could spend their lives solving crimes.

My client's cat eventually passed on, and the client moved away. I still have several of "The Cat Who" books she lent to me.

I had better read them soon. I may find other medical miracles within those pages.

27. Mrs. M.

When I first began doing house calls in earnest as a part-time job aside from my employment at an animal hospital, I received a call from the elderly Mrs. M.

She was very concerned about her two Siamese cats, Mookie and Pookie, who, as the breed goes, were middle-aged at 15. One of them had "irregularity."

I examined each one in turn, then lined the bathroom floor with newspaper and gently administered an enema. Success came immediately, and I had a new and devoted client. Little did I know this would be a chronic issue, necessitating many visits. As they aged, Mookie and Pookie had many problems, and Mrs. M. would constantly call me. The thing was, when she got started talking on the phone, she never stopped. Finally, in the background, my husband would yell, "Fire! Get out of the house!" and she would finally hang up. I never had to utter a word when she called, as her conversation consisted of one run-on sentence.

Mrs. M. lived on top of a mountain, so getting to her house was no easy feat in the middle of winter. I would brace myself in my car as it trudged up the hill, praying I would arrive intact. With Mrs. M., there were no excuses. She called and put on her most mournful tone, and before I knew it I was on my way.

Her husband had dementia and could not remember if or when the cats had been fed, so she would leave large signs on all of the doors telling him what to do. The most interesting thing about Mr. M. was that he was always at the piano, playing old show tunes by heart. Though he could hardly even remember his own name, his music memory remained intact until he died. He provided beautiful melodies on his piano for my listening pleasure, while I treated the cats. For many years, I took care of Mrs. M.'s cats until they finally died, but I will always remember her and Mookie and Pookie.

28. Celebrities

Occasionally I would get a call from a person who was the housekeeper or the assistant of a celebrity asking me to do a house call. Once it involved a Russian blue cat.

I came over quite star-struck, but after speaking with the well-known person, I realized that the owner was just a nice, normal person. As I examined the cat, she told jokes and stories. I recommended a dental cleaning for the cat, and the next thing I knew, I was picking up Melvin to bring him in to the office. When I brought him back to his home later that day, the reception was warm and welcoming.

One day at this celebrity's house, I was looking for Melvin, who was usually in the bathroom for the exam. Slightly chagrined that I could not find him, I decided to use the separate toilet, which was beckoning to me with its heated seat that pops up when one is nearby. I entered and closed the door.

While sitting there, I noticed a big stack of books. In the middle of my "activity," I overheard my assistant talking to someone right in the bathroom, outside the toilet door. I quickly finished up and exited the toilet, and there was my client! Embarrassed and flushed (no pun intended), I proceeded to wash my hands and examine my patient, whom she was holding in her arms.

Through the years I have had to see Melvin on many occasions, most recently for his inflammatory bowel disease. I sometimes find him sitting on the big bed, watching his owner on television, and probably feeling comforted by seeing her image on the screen.

29. Getting lost

One of the hardest things about doing a house call in an unfamiliar area is finding the destination. Before GPS became commonplace, I would interview potential employees by showing them an address of a house call. Then I would ask them to find it for me on the map. I brought atlases to the interview, including the eight counties that we serve. Some candidates would hold the map upside down and sideways to try to make sense of it. Others would look at the index and find the key to figuring out a particular location. They would approach the problem with fervor, and still come up short. Still others would admit they never learned how to read a map.

Then came the GPS. My car had one built in, and "she" guided us to the house calls. Her voice sounded like "The Exorcist," and she occasionally had us going down a one-way street the wrong way. If the weather was inclement or the terrain mountainous, the signal would be lost, and we would be driving around in circles hoping for a sign of which way to go. If there was a road block, we could not tell the GPS person to create another route, as the voice kept redirecting us back to that site.

This was a big problem. It slowed us down, made us late for subsequent house calls, and made us cranky. Later I abandoned "The Exorcist" for a Garman, and then the maps app on the iphone. I still find that nothing is 100 percent perfect.

In the process of giving over my voyage to a voice on the radio, I feel I have lost an innate ability to navigate and in some ways have lost my sense of direction.

One example of these traveling woes was the day my assistant and I embarked on a trip to a town several miles away, in an urban center full of traffic snares, highways, and bridges. We finally arrived at the house call to examine a cat. We were behind schedule by then and a bit flustered by the trip.

One look at our feline patient and we knew all was well. I examined my patient and performed the needed services and then gathered my belongings and left. Later that day, at another house call, I realized that my fluid bag was missing. Calling the previous house calls to see if it were there, I finally learned where we had left it: in the house that was so hard to find.

I worked out a plan with the owner to meet in a location midway between my base and her house. I sat in the parking lot waiting for her like someone waiting to hook up with a drug dealer. Then she appeared and returned my bright orange fluid bag, which was a sight for sore eyes, and glowed like the sun. I got up and went on my way, very grateful and a little embarrassed.

30. The Elvis family reunion

At the veterinary clinic we used to have a client and benefactor who was an angel to the animals. She would rescue whomever she could and find homes for them. One day she brought in a pregnant cat. The litter was born at the hospital just around the time a friend of mine was looking for a cat for her family.

My friend's daughter picked out one of the kittens and named her Elvis. Elvis went on to have one litter of four kittens before being spayed.

Out of the four kittens, only Sarah is still alive. The others met their maker while adventuring outside.

I noted that Sarah was a survivor after 12 years of going outdoors and having the gene for adventure.

She managed to avoid the cars, trucks, coyotes, and bears. But Elvis, the mama cat, is still around, too. It had been a teenage pregnancy, so they are only six months apart. They live near each other, so for all I know, they meet every once in a while for lunch and to reminisce.

31. Surgeries in the car

It was 7:30 a.m. on the first Wednesday of November. It was my surgery day at the animal hospital. I arrived at Ms. S.'s house, cloaked in heavy clothes with a tranquilizer injection ready to go. There, in her bathroom, hidden behind the litter box and stacks of canned Fancy Feast, was my patient. Millie needed a dental procedure with extractions. The only problem was that she was feral, so I sneaked up behind her and plunged the syringe into her rump before she could react.

In a short while, I heard her growling subside, so it was time to gently place her in the carrier, and off to work I went. I had the surgery technicians prepare for the dentistry. This entailed blood work, an EKG, and an IV catheter, then intubating her and placing her on inhalation anesthesia and oxygen. Once the fluids were running, we were ready to begin.

Cats normally have 30 teeth, but Millie had only 15 remaining in her mouth, and two of those were coming out. She did well and was placed back in her carrier before she woke up, with the catheter out and no bandages to remove. This would have been impossible in a feral cat. Later, the owner picked her up and took her home. Millie was happy to be rid of those rotten teeth.

32. No Medicare for cats

Mrs. N. was in her late 80s and lived on the third floor of a house, but she was able negotiate the stairs more quickly than a woman half her age and looked like a sprite as she descended them.

She had a 14-year-old cat named Nancy who had always loved to eat. When I first met her, the cat weighed 22 pounds and was always hungry. She had the frame of a 10-pound cat, so she would waddle around the house hardly able to get away when we chased her for the exam. Mrs. N. could not put her in the bathroom, so we always had to look for her and round her up.

As time went on, I put Nancy on a weight-reduction diet, and she began to lose the weight. Mrs. N. was very diligent with her feedings and never let her have a single morsel more than I recommended. I was always worried that Nancy would develop diabetes, as overweight older cats were more likely to get this disease.

The years went by, and Nancy achieved her goal weight of 13 pounds. Then the strangest thing began to happen. She started losing *more* weight. Her appetite was still very good, so I thought it might be hyperthyroidism, which older cats often get. This disease causes a benign tumor to grow on the thyroid gland, which secretes thyroid hormone causing an increased metabolic rate. This would make a cat eat more yet still lose weight.

The treatment for this is medication to reduce the thyroid hormone secretion, iodine-deficient diet, surgery, or a radioactive iodine injection. We tested Nancy, and she was indeed positive for hyperthyroidism. We started her on the medication and noticed that her white blood cells dropped to below normal.

This could be one of the side effects, so we had to stop the medicine. Instead, we put her on the dietary option.

The cat was doing well for a while and then stopped eating altogether and started hiding in the closet. Now the question was: Did she not like the diet or was she ill with another problem? The exam did not show any abdominal masses or heart murmurs, but she was dehydrated. We gave her subcutaneous fluids, an anti-vomiting medicine, an antibiotic, and a vitamin injection. Mrs. N. was telling me she was having company the following week and could not bear it if the cat were sick. We took blood and urine tests and waited for the results.

Unfortunately, we discovered that Nancy was suffering from chronic renal (kidney) failure and was rapidly deteriorating.

In vet school I had done my senior seminar on "Chronic Renal Failure in the Cat." This is most often seen in the geriatric cat. I see how an animal ages gracefully and then one day suddenly falls very ill. I described the clinical signs, the diagnosis, and the treatment of this problem.

Chronic kidney failure is a progressive disease, which starts off with subtle signs. The previously hungry cat may become a picky eater. The cat who you never saw drinking from the water bowl is now hanging out there and taking frequent drinks. The litter box may become very wet. The cat may become sleepy and not as active as he used to be. He may seem to be a bit grouchy and less friendly and playful. These signs are vague and difficult to match up with chronic kidney failure. Many other diseases can cause increased thirst and urination, decreased appetite, and lethargy, but in an older cat, my first suspicion is kidney disease. Blood work and urinalysis can confirm this diagnosis.

There are five stages in the IRIS (International Renal Interest Society) system. Nancy had rapidly progressed to stage five. The previous blood work a few months before had been normal. This could possibly be influenced by other factors such as dehydration and infection.

Cats are unusual in that once fluids and other supportive care are given, some can improve to some degree and remain in a stable condition for several months to years. This disease is an insidious one, and it sometimes seems to come out of the blue in an otherwise healthy animal. The causes of chronic kidney failure in the cat are numerous, but once it occurs, it is like discovering a building that has burned down and trying to find out what caused the fire. Some of the functions of the kidney are to filter the blood, remove wastes, control the body's fluid balance, and regulate the balance of electrolytes.

After trying intravenous fluids in the hospital for a few days, there was no improvement, so Mrs. N. had to put Nancy to sleep. The only thing that would have helped was dialysis or a renal transplant, neither of which Mrs. N could afford.

There is no Medicare for cats.

33. My scale never lies.

Melba is a 22-year-old, British, short-haired, female cat who has high blood pressure, hyperthyroidism, and kidney disease. She has very caring owners who watch her like a hawk and can tell if she has lost an ounce. They keep a close eye on her, having me come over to take periodic blood pressures, weights, and blood tests. Melba "complains" during these procedures, but right after, she is back at the food dish as though nothing had happened.

This time it appeared she had lost some weight. The blood pressure was normal on the medication, and her thyroid level was well controlled, but just two weeks earlier she had weighed a pound more. We decided it might have been the scale at the hospital. Some of the scales tend to put on an extra pound, and that can make a big difference in a small cat. The owners, being so watchful about her weight, were not comforted in knowing the scale might have been off. She had also been at the hospital four weeks earlier and was the same weight as she was when I saw her. That was a different scale. So is this cat losing weight? Only time will tell, when I come over next time and reweigh her on *my* scale. My scale never lies.

34. Oleo

Oleo is a 17-year-old spayed cat with owners who dote on her endlessly. They take excellent care of her and were heartbroken when she developed chronic kidney failure. She did well on daily subcutaneous fluids, blood pressure medications and a special diet to preserve kidney function. I would check on her every month or two to see how she was doing. I would weigh her, check her heart and lungs, feel her kidneys and bladder, take her blood pressure, and collect blood and urine. She was one of the fortunate ones, maintaining satisfactory health despite her illness, and the owners were happy to keep it that way.

One day she was not acting normally, licking her rump and hissing. She was brought into the clinic, and it was discovered that she had an anal gland abscess. It was lanced and drained under inhalation anesthesia, after which she was feeling much better.

The reason for the hissing and hiding had been that she was in pain, but in older cats, there are many sources of pain. These can be arthritis, bladder pain, and pain from dental disease.

I routinely recommend arthritis medication to decrease pain and also that the owner cut a hole in the litter box so the cat does not have to climb too high. We have an arsenal of pain medications for older cats, and we should not hesitate to use them. We want to give each cat the best quality of life he can have.

35. Cats don't read the book.

Mrs. Q. calls me often to check on her cat, Popo, a female domestic shorthair with a tendency to lick the fur off of her thighs, forelegs, and belly. I ran several tests to determine the cause, and they came back negative. I explained that the best way to resolve the licking would be to feed an exclusively hypoallergenic diet, and Mrs. Q. did that, but she always added some tuna as a treat a few times a week. This lessened any good effects of the diet, but Popo looked forward to her tuna, so there was no negotiation. As the cat aged, she had frequent check-ups. Mrs. Q. wanted to be sure to catch any problem before it became serious. The check-ups were her way of trying to ensure her cat's future, but sometimes cats get sick despite all of our efforts.

I would routinely examine Popo in a spacious bathroom, full of Mrs. Q.'s perfumes. There were over 25 bottles of various fragrances, from Coco Chanel to Bulgaria's Jasmine Noir to The One.

One day, Mrs. Q. noticed that the litter box was soaked and Popo had started drinking a lot and vomiting as well. Popo was still active and playful and eating well. I began to ponder the possibilities. In this 14-year-old cat, high on the list were diabetes, kidney disease, hyperthyroidism, and pancreatitis. A tumor in the intestinal tract or elsewhere also had to be considered. Or, it could be nothing.

I examined the cat and noted a weight loss of five ounces since the last visit six months before. I listened to the heart and the lungs and felt the abdomen. I did an ophthalmic exam, looked into the mouth, and felt the neck for a thyroid nodule. I took the blood pressure and blood and urine samples. The blood glucose was elevated, so diabetes may have been the problem. The full lab work would be done to confirm it, as well as a urinalysis and subsequent blood glucose testing.

Sometimes cats get stress hyperglycemia, so if this is the case, another blood sugar may be normal; that is why we never base a diagnosis of diabetes on one blood sugar level in the cat. In addition, the cat had high blood pressure, and medication would be recommended if this were repeatable. Blood pressure can go up from stress also.

In cats, if diabetes is diagnosed within six months of its onset and treated with insulin, remission is possible in up to 50 percent of the cases. Diabetes in the cat has become an epidemic. The middle-aged to older cat is most often affected. There are many factors involved, but the cat is sometimes overweight and may be on a high carbohydrate diet. Treatment with insulin resolves the signs, but the owner must be diligent with monitoring water intake, urination, and appetite and administer insulin twice a day. Blood sugars are also measured either at home or at the clinic.

As soon as I mentioned diabetes, Mrs. Q. began to tear up, asking what she might have done to cause it and what she might have done differently to prevent it, as if there was a specific cause that could have been avoided.

I remembered an article I had read in the New York Times about medical reversal. Many people are told to eat a certain diet to help stabilize blood sugar in diabetes. However, findings reveal that these measures do nothing to increase the lifespan of an individual. With this in mind, I thought of Popo. She had the genetic make-up that led her to this day. It was not evident that it could have been avoided. The only thing in our control is weight management, but at 12 pounds, Popo was not considered obese, so this condition was probably predetermined long before it became an overt illness, and no amount of exams and blood tests was going to change that.

36. Help! We're locked in the bathroom!

One day I was asked to see two cats who lived in a spacious home in a gated community. I entered the house and found it to be like a museum, with massive hallways full of gigantic paintings. The owner led us to the bathroom in her son's room, where the cats were.

We entered, closed the door, and set out to examine each cat. When we were finished, we packed up and were about to leave, but we could not open the door; it was jammed. No matter how hard we tried, it would not budge. We banged on it loudly to try to attract attention, but no one could hear us as the residents and housekeeper were on the opposite side of the house. We looked out of the bathroom window and saw a beautiful pool and a large backyard. We knocked on the window and again were not heard.

My technician and I looked at each other, puzzled that we could not figure out how to get out of the bathroom. The cats just sat there watching us, seemingly amused. We had no cell phones at the time, and the only thing we could do was wait. Finally, the housekeeper heard our knocking and released us. We had never been so glad to leave a bathroom as we were that day.

37. The cat always wins!

Whenever I go on a cat house call, I always instruct the owner to have the animal in the bathroom or a small room with a large towel outside the room before I arrive. I use the towel to prevent the cat from escaping as I enter the room. Once inside, I secure my patient and call my technician in with my medical bags and scale.

Unfortunately, many people do not listen to my request. Sometimes they put the towel *in* the bathroom instead of outside. Other times they choose a room with a couch or a bed, where the cat can easily hide. Worst of all are those who do not put the cat in any room at all. One day I had two clients in a row who did just that.

The first client, Mr. T, had three cats who go outside. Upon entering the house, I noticed the front door was wide open, as a painter was working there. This was a bad sign. I wondered if the cats were even in the house.

Mr. T. did not know where they were. First he checked the basement and found no cats. Then he went to the second floor. My technician and I stood on either side of the bottom landing to prevent each cat from escaping. Mr. T. brought Daffodil into the bathroom, and we did the exam, weighed her, and gave her the annual vaccinations.

Next it was Great Guy's turn.

Finally, it was Lily's turn. By some miracle, Mr. T. had been able to pick each one up, bring him or her downstairs to the bathroom, and have us do our thing.

Our next house call was to a new client, Mrs. X. She explained on the phone that her cat, Helena, was very fearful, afraid of strangers, and refused to get into a carrier. I told her we could come, but we would need to have the cat in the bathroom or a similar small room before our arrival.

We arrived and found that the cat was loose in the house. The 87-year-old owner had tried for hours to get Helena into the laundry room, but the cat was having no part of it.

Cats are much better at escaping capture than we are at catching them. As I watched Mrs. X. kneel on the floor to look under the credenza, trying to coax Helena out, I heard the cat meow in return, as if to say, "You have got to be kidding!"

We finally left, unable to see the cat that day. So in the end, when it is cat versus man, the cat always wins.

38. The cat who could not breathe

We went to see a cat who was on medication for hyperthyroidism and needed a blood test to check her levels. The last time she went to the office, her breathing had been so labored that the doctor had become very concerned. He had given her a very guarded prognosis and recommended a house call for subsequent blood tests.

The cat lived in a plumber's office, and as soon as we entered the room, we were struck by the overwhelming odor of cigarette smoke. I commented that it would help if the cat were not in the same room as the smoke as she already had respiratory difficulties, and this would just make them worse. The man replied, "My boss has been smoking all of his life, and at 67, he isn't going to change." I recommended getting an air filter and then took the blood test.

Though her breathing was labored through the test, as soon as we finished, she quickly recovered and hid under a chair. This was much less traumatic than bringing her to the office. I was sorry that I could not convince the owners to keep her away from the cigarette smoke that was resulting in poor air quality.

Sometimes I can only educate. I cannot dictate.

39. Mr. C. and Le Pew

I first met Mr. C. when he called me to examine Le Pew, his middle-aged tabby, and to clip his nails. I would go there for wellness visits, and all was well for a while. Mr. C. was a lawyer by day but also a singer in a musical group specializing in political satire. He used a wheelchair, but he moved as quickly as the next person, and did not let this disability stop him in any way.

The years passed, and Le Pew started having some problems. The blood work showed he had become diabetic. We started him on insulin, and he did very well. He went into remission twice and then came out of it, so he had to be monitored very closely.

Mr. C. was very good at noticing the smallest changes in Le Pew's' behavior. He would almost know what the blood sugar level was before I checked it. He also had many theories about why it was hard to regulate his cat. The insulin was too old, or it was too new, the dose was too high, or it was too low, Le Pew had had too much to eat, or had not had enough.

Whatever the case, Le Pew spent more than five years as a happy diabetic. Then one day he started getting intestinal issues, then kidney issues, then a tumor in his lungs. It was harder to keep him in the right zone with respect to his blood sugar, and, consequently, his quality of life began to suffer. One day it was time to say goodbye to Le Pew. I euthanized him in the comfort of his own home next to the one he loved the most, Mr. C.

Mr. C.'s relationship with his cat was one of intense affection and respect. The cat will be missed for a very long time, and I will miss coming over and examining him and watching how the two of them related to each other. It was a very special bond indeed.

40. Don't touch my food dish!

I often go to a house call with multiple cats. It is somewhat easy to add another cat to an established cat household, as they use a litter box and are fairly independent. People are able to go away for a day or two and leave a big bowl of dry food and plenty of fresh water for these pets. This is not possible with a dog.

Before a new cat enters the home, he or she is checked for any diseases or parasites and given a healthy diagnosis. People are usually willing to do this. The one thing they overlook is that sometimes cats do not play nicely together. In the wild, cats have individual territories and protect them by fighting if they see an approaching cat. They also stalk their prey and eat alone, not with their fellow cats beside them eating their own rewards.

In a house, they are in an unnatural environment. They are asked to cooperate and use that little rectangular box filled with clay to do their business, possibly with another cat or dog or human looking on. They are asked to get along with the other residents and share food and resources. Many simply refuse.

On one such visit, there were five cats in a modest-sized home. They often fought and occasionally had bite wounds. They were strictly indoor cats but were also surrounded by outside neighborhood cats. The odds were against them as far as becoming pleasant and charming. Each day they had to reassert themselves in the dominance chain, and stress levels were high.

I examined three of these cats and found them all to be a bit overweight, very nervous, and unsettled. The calmest one betrayed himself by having the fastest heart rate—a sign of anxiety. They were all breathing heavily, and they all sported battle wounds. It looked to me as if they were suffering from chronic stress and overeating from worry about having their food stolen by the other cats. The owners tried to keep the most aggressive male away from the others, but the rest of the cats had their own intraspecific aggression issues. There were simply too many asocial cats living under one roof. Would they ever get along? I recommended behavioral conditioning between two at a time and the use of anti-aggression and anti-anxiety medications. The conditioning places two of the cats in carriers 20 feet apart, gradually moving them closer until the owner sees a reaction and then goes back a step. Then they are fed with one out of the carrier, again 20 feet apart. Gradually they are both fed out of the carriers, and, little by little, they are fed in closer proximity.

This is no easy task, and it may take months to achieve a truce, but it can work and may lead to a more harmonious cat family. We shall see.

41. Unusual gifts

Many times when I go on a house call, I come away with not only a blood sample and a stool sample, but also a small gift. One older woman whose cat needed an exam gave me a can of sardines that she claimed was delicious.

Another client gave me a CD of French opera singers when he found out that I studied French.

Another client, who had once been a famous Broadway actress but was now in her 90s, gave me a giant throw blanket. I have received special teas, fresh-baked chocolate chip cookies, beautiful crocheted afghans, a book of guinea pigs acting out "Pride and Prejudice," a plaque saying "Cats Are People Too," another plaque saying "Don't Bite Off More Than You Can Chew," and still another saying "Cats leave paw prints on your heart."

At the holidays, some of my clients would send gifts. Once anyone knew I loved frogs, the gifts came pouring in with a frog theme. These included frog purses, frog pins, frog earrings, frog clocks, frog lamps and frog candles. My whole wall unit is full of frog tchotchkes. I also receive a wonderful, big box of cookies each year from the same client.

There is no forgetting Mrs. U. She was a benefactor for the animal hospital, having helped my boss when he had started out there. She rescued many animals and would bring them in for help.

Every holiday season she brought the entire staff gifts, tailored to each staff member. She bought me gift certificates to Kohls and Wild Birds Unlimited, sweaters, jewelry, and outerwear. She loved us all and showed it at the holidays. She was an angel, both to the animals she saved and to us. Although she has passed on, these gifts keep her in our hearts.

42. Mr. Scrappy and the nose tumor

I had been asked to do a house call on a cat who had developed a very large tumor on his nose. It was analyzed and found to be a fibrosarcoma. This was a very malignant and invasive mass, and removal would be difficult. This procedure was to be followed by further treatment, such as radiation.

Due to its location, the mass was inoperable, so the little cat did not have a bright future. When I first examined him, he was a scrappy fellow and not too friendly, but what stood out was this ping pong ball on top of his nose. It was ulcerated and bleeding.

I prescribed pain medications, and a week later the owner was ready to say goodbye. The tumor had doubled in size in one week. It was time to put Scrappy to sleep. My technician reached for him under the couch, and despite his ornery attitude, he allowed himself to be brought out for me to give the sedative before we euthanized him. It was as if he knew the time had come. He was ready.

Chapter Three

Rabbits

43. Quincy, the rabbit gardener

The small, brown rabbit had the entire back room of the house to himself. He merrily ran around, climbing onto stacks of shelves to get a better view of the outdoors. The owner's favorite pastime was gardening, and she would let Quincy accompany her as she raked, weeded, and planted.

One day she noticed he was not feeling well, so she called me for a house call. I examined Quincy and was surprised at what I discovered: Throughout his body were lumps and ulcers, one right on his scrotum. These were cuterebra, or bots, the larvae of botflies. Quincy had to go to the hospital for surgery.

I took him to my clinic, anesthetized him, and prepared the sites. I gently opened each bot location and removed the bot, then cleaned and flushed the area and let it heal.

During the gardening, Quincy had picked up the bots while he roamed across the soil. Bots cause toxins to release if they are lacerated, so removal must be done very carefully. I also performed a castration and a scrotal ablation. Quincy did well and had no more bots.

I told the owner, "No more gardening with Quincy!"

44. Poetic justice

I was at a local pet megastore treating a guinea pig with a fungal infection. As I was finishing up and writing up my chart, I was eager to meet my daughter whom I had dropped off next door at the supermarket to do the food shopping. I was packing up when a store manager ran to the wellness room with a panting rabbit. He had been left for adoption, but was in dire straits.

He had been left outdoors where the temperature was 90 degrees and had developed heat stroke. The rabbit's breathing was fast and labored, and he was in a state of collapse. I took his temperature, which was 106 degrees, confirming my fears.

I requested some cool, wet cloths to place over his head and trunk, did a physical exam, and administered fluids. Once the rabbit was stable, I met my daughter at the car parked in the supermarket lot, and we went on our way.

This incident happened in early June, and it reminded me of another early June day when I was 14. I was spending the day in Manhattan with friends, and my mom decided to clean the rabbit cage, which contained two bunnies. She brought the cage into the garden, placed it in the shade, and set about her chores, with the cage's cleaning on her short list.

The list wasn't short enough, however, because when she returned outside to the garden, she was shocked to find both rabbits dead. The sun had shifted and was directly over the cage. Since rabbits cannot tolerate direct sunlight or temperatures higher than 84 degrees, they had developed heat stroke that led to their demise.

So it is poetic justice that, all these years later, on the same June day, I was at the right place at the right time and was able to save a bunny from the same fate.

45. Popsy, the bunny

Poor Popsy started having problems at the age of 6. This is considered old in rabbit years. He began to drink and eat less. He was also producing fewer fecal pellets. The owner, Mrs. C., and her 12-year-old son were very concerned.

They brought Popsy in for an exam. I found him to be a bit lethargic and noticed he had lost 10 percent of his body weight. He was dehydrated and had a doughy abdomen. I worried he had developed gastric stasis. This is a common condition in rabbits when their diet is low in fiber, or they have a hairball in the stomach, or other factors such as little exercise or stress. Dietary fiber encourages normal gastrointestinal processes.

Gastric stasis is very serious. The food just sits in the stomach and does not move out to the small intestines. This leads to dehydration, scant stool, lethargy, and pain. The rabbit may have not eaten in days and have large, dough-like stomach contents. The gut sounds are silent, and the temperature may be low. Treatment includes giving subcutaneous or intravenous fluids, hydrating the stomach contents, motility agents, and pain reducers. Antibiotics are used to decrease bacterial overgrowth. A critical-care diet is fed by syringe.

For Popsy, treatment led to great improvement. I had Mrs. C. and her son check the stool production, appetite, and thirst every day. At the next visit, Popsy had regained the weight he had lost, was eating well, and was well-hydrated. Mrs. C.'s son collected the stool the rabbit had produced in the last day and brought it in for me to see.

From then on, I would see Popsy regularly to check his weight and listen for gut sounds. Mrs. C.'s son diligently brought in a plastic bag containing each and every fecal pellet that Popsy had produced in the last 24 hours. Mrs. C. learned how to administer fluids at home, and she gave the medications I prescribed to keep him healthy. I doubt that Popsy would be doing so well without the care his owners gave him. But he is only a "hare" away from becoming sick again if he eats the wrong thing or does not get enough water.

46. The new bunny

The owner called about a new pet she had just adopted. It was a male rabbit who had been left behind by a neighbor who was moving. Since he was black and white, the family had named him Oreo. I came into the house and was greeted by this lop-eared rabbit who had the run of the place, prancing around the living room, pooping as he went. He was gentle until someone tried to pick him up. Then he turned into a frightened prisoner who wanted to escape anyone's grasp.

I placed him on the floor between my legs and gently began to examine him. Then I cut his very long nails. I went over diet and husbandry with the owner, how to litter train the rabbit even when outside of the cage, and proper rabbit-proofing techniques. I noted there were a lot of electronics and wires in the living room and asked the owner if she could remove them, but she said she always watches him.

I know from my own rabbit who had chewed right through my computer printer cord that it only takes about three seconds for them to go through a wire. If it were connected to live electricity, this could result in mouth burns or worse. If the phone rang or the teakettle boiled, that would create enough time to allow for damage.

The other thing I noticed was that the front entrance to the house had just one door, and the rabbit was very close to it. How long before he ventured out into the lush, green lawn to sample the delicious grass? I recommended that they get in touch with the House Rabbit Society, a group that has a lot of information to help rabbit owners raise their rabbits safely and happily.

They also had a Boston terrier, who came into the house from the yard and ran over to greet us, not paying much attention to Oreo. The dog and the rabbit got along very well. The owner's son thought it was because they were both black and white, so they felt related.

Chapter Four

All Creatures Great...

47. Pigs as pets

In vet school, we learned about the different breeds of pigs and all of the diseases they can get. We learned their anatomy and physiology and were exposed to pigs that were treated there. We also saw breeding pigs with several piglets in tow.

Potbellied pigs came into vogue as household pets in the 1980s. They are smaller than standard pigs and can be litter-trained. While at a veterinary conference in New Orleans, I met a physician who owned a pig. He was standing next to me in line at Paul Prudhomme's restaurant, and we sat next to each other at one of the long tables.

He described the Yorkshire pig who shared his home, sat and watched television, and knew how to open the refrigerator. There was even an article written about their relationship in Newsweek. He said his pig was human-like and very smart.

Years later I thought about getting a pet pig. So I took a trip to "pig country" with my daughter and one of my favorite technicians. Outside of a farm we saw a sign stating they had baby pigs for sale, and we stopped to take a look. We parked the car and walked into the barn, where a young man greeted us.

I told him I was thinking of buying a baby pig. He said they went for 10 cents a pound. He showed us a little baby, which I held and fell in love with, thinking of Wilbur in "Charlotte's Web."

Then the young man warned me, "When he gets to be an adult, this is what he will look like," and he pointed to a pig that was several feet long and weighed more than 750 pounds. I took one look at him and tripped and fell down. Knowing that I was not able to accommodate such a giant pet, I thanked him and we left, somewhat discouraged. That doesn't mean I won't reconsider it in the future!

48. The "big dog" lover

One of my clients loves big dogs. When I first did a house call for her, I examined two St. Bernards and one Newfoundland; later she bought a fourth dog, a little shih tzu, who seemed to be the boss.

The large dogs were as sweet as pie, allowing me to examine them, poking and probing, without so much as a whimper. After their exams, they would quickly retreat to their kennels, where they felt safe.

The dogs were allowed in the big, back room of the house and had access to a large backyard with bushes surrounding it. The only dog who had the run of the house was Boris, the little one.

Year after year, one of the big dogs would test positive for Lyme or another tick-borne disease, despite having been vaccinated and put on flea and tick preventatives. This particular dog loved to walk the perimeter of the yard, where the bushes were. She would go as far as she could into the foliage, making her an easy target for any ticks residing there.

New Jersey is one of the worst states in the country for Lyme disease. Deer are very abundant; they carry the Ixodes tick, which transmits it. We see one in four dogs with either Lyme or another tick-related illness. Signs of Lyme can range from lameness to fever to just being lethargic. In some dogs, Lyme disease can affect the kidneys, causing inflammation. We don't usually see the bull's-eye lesion that is found in humans in the early stages.

In addition to vaccination, tick prevention should always be used. Lyme vaccinations target the Lyme organism both in the tick and in the dog. At certain times of the year, the ticks are so numerous that despite all of this, one tick may still slip through the cracks. Therefore, it is important to remain vigilant about tick control and careful when going into the woods or even one's own backyard.

Lyme disease in dogs reflects a similar situation for their owners. The dog is considered a sentinel. I always tell an owner that there are ticks around and they should use caution. If they are gardening or doing yard work, I advise that they cover up well and do a tick check on themselves regularly. In this way the veterinary community can help people to protect themselves from becoming infected.

49. Great Danes

Great Danes are wonderful pets, but as with any purebred dog, they are predisposed to certain maladies. One great Dane patient suffered from arthritis at a young age due to his large bones.

Another developed allergies, causing itchy feet and face that I treated with baths and antihistamines. Sometimes a food component is responsible, and a hypoallergenic diet is fed for at least eight weeks to see if that helps. I have one such patient who eats only a raw diet, so a food trial is not possible. These allergies lead to hair loss, scaling, and chronic itching. Sometimes secondary infections occur, and it becomes a life-long challenge.

The biggest and most serious problem is bloat, which is more common in this breed. The stomach of the dog is not attached to the body wall, and when full of food, it can rotate on its axis. This is more likely if a dog runs a lot right after eating a big meal.

The prognosis for bloat is extremely guarded. When it leads to gastric torsion, the dog needs emergency veterinary care and aggressive fluid therapy. Once the dog is stable, surgical correction can be performed. During this procedure, the stomach is de-rotated, and then tacked down to the body wall to prevent it from happening again.

Any dog can get bloat. Large dogs are more susceptible, and many dog owners request a preventive tack-down be done before their dog can come to any harm.

I first learned about bloat from my saxophone teacher when I was 15. He had owned great Danes through the years, and one of them had developed bloat. He said the dog was running around after he had eaten a large meal, and the stomach had turned around and caused a bloat and torsion. No food could enter or exit, and this caused it to dilate with gas and toxins. These entered the bloodstream and poisoned the dog, resulting in his death. My teacher was very sad and determined never to let this happen to one of his dogs again.

Little did he know that he was educating me about more than jazz syncopation at my music lessons.

Chapter Five

...And Small

50. Sharing ideas

Many pet megastore personnel help me when I treat their animals. Some have special training and love to share their thoughts with me. One day while I was examining my 15th hamster with wet tail—a disease that causes severe diarrhea and dehydration and often leads to death—one small-animal specialist surmised that this problem seemed more prevalent as the seasons change. I agreed, though, truthfully, wet tail is a syndrome with many causes, including bacteria, viruses, parasites, stress, climate, humidity, transport, age, etc. They either get better or they don't.

When I was 11, I had been raising more than 20 hamsters. Occasionally I would witness a wet tail. The hamster was hunched, walked like a 100-year-old person, had become weak, and suffered from severe diarrhea. At that time I did a lot of reading and discovered that hamsters get thiamine deficiency and need supplemental Vitamin B1, so I started giving them enriched bread, and they got better. That is why I give all my wet tail patients a Vitamin B injection and recommend adding warm oatmeal to their diet. I recently attended a lecture on rodent medicine, and wet tail came up, but no one said anything about Vitamin B. I knew that it worked.

51. Hamster disorders

At a pet megastore I examined a short-haired teddy bear hamster with no use of his hind legs due to a terrible fight with a cage mate. Hamsters can become very aggressive to their cage mates when they are mature, and the best way to prevent this sort of thing is to separate them when they are 4 months old. This hamster was permanently injured, and there would be a very rocky road ahead. I imagined building a mini-cart for him, but realized his internal injuries were too severe to treat.

Another type of hamster I see at the store is the Djungarian hamster. These little guys are hearty and never get wet tail. They weigh only 40 grams but act like little Napoleons. They are not friendly nor do they enjoy being handled. One hamster was found with a swollen right front leg, and I brought her to the hospital. I gave her a pre-anesthetic, which sedated her heavily. She had radiographs and then inhalation anesthesia while I made an incision on her tiny leg, flushed the area, cultured it, and sutured the wound closed. Post-op and still groggy, she turned into the sweetest hamster ever and allowed me to feed her critical-care diet by syringe once she was awake. By day's end, every technician wanted to take her home.

She returned to the wellness room of the pet store with no permanent home in her future. I eventually adopted her, naming her Beatrice after a favorite jazz standard, and gave her a good home until she passed on several years later.

She never lost that Napoleonic complex.

52. The gerbil without a tail

On my travels as a house call vet I see many different species of animals. In one case I had to treat a male gerbil at a pet megastore with a tail injury. In the cage next to him in the wellness room was a female hamster that I had just examined, and I had not yet put the cover back on the tank.

As I prepared to examine the gerbil's tail, he jumped out of my hand, darted 12 inches into the air, and landed in the hamster's cage.

She was in her little house, nesting, and when she saw and heard the gerbil's grand entrance, she screamed at the top of her lungs. I could almost make out the words, "Get out of my house!" The intruder was quickly retrieved, sedated, and the tail amputated. He recovered nicely, no worse for the experience in his unfriendly neighbor's abode.

53. The guinea pig whisperer

Ever since I got my first call from Mrs. L. I knew she was a guinea pig devotee. She loved her little guys and tried to do whatever she could to help them when they were ill. She has a small graveyard in her backyard, where her deceased pets are buried.

One day she brought one into the clinic and had to leave him there for supportive care as he was suffering from a severe infection. She would visit every day and would cry as she held him. She let the tears fall on him, and she said they had healing powers. The guinea pig eventually improved and went home, thus reinforcing her theory.

Most recently she returned from a trip abroad and noticed that one of her guinea pigs was breathing loudly. She called me at once to arrange a house call. The next day I visited Jimmy and diagnosed a respiratory infection. I gave him a Vitamin C injection and dispensed antibiotics. Guinea pigs have a requirement for Vitamin C, as they are unable to manufacture their own. Therefore, if they do not get it from food and other sources, they can develop scurvy. They have this in common with humans. With a Vitamin C deficiency, a guinea pig will develop respiratory infections, fever, diarrhea, decreased appetite, have pain when walking, develop bleeding gums, and other symptoms.

When Mrs. L. came near him, Jimmy started grunting and giving a low whistle, one of many vocalizations guinea pigs emit to convey joy. Luckily, Mrs. L. is an astute owner, able to tell when one of her pet pals is sick long before anyone else could.

54. The neighborhood pet store with the personal touch

For more than 15 years I have made house calls at The Brookdale Pet Center in Bloomfield, New Jersey. The store has been in business since 1995, and it has an old-fashioned hometown feel. Each staff member knows each customer by name. Their mission statement reads: "to serve our community and to provide our patrons and animals with the products, knowledge and service for a happier and healthier life." They invite speakers to lecture on the benefits of various diets for dogs and cats. They foster animals that are up for adoption and have moved away from buying animals from a warehouse distributor.

One of their fosters is Master Splinter, who is an Agouti fancy rat. He was originally ordered for a customer who never picked him up. Within three weeks he became too large for the potential owner to feed to his snake, so the staff decided to keep him. He is affectionate and playful and personifies all of the great qualities of rats.

Another example is a bearded dragon who was boarded and left at the pet shop due to a divorce. The staff built a superior enclosure for him with all of the comforts of home, and he is going to be adopted shortly.

They also work with a guinea pig rescue organization and try to find homes for these critters, a noble enterprise. The guinea pigs they formerly received from the distributor were usually ill with skin or respiratory ailments.

The birds in the pet shop are tame, and many were hand-raised. The staff spends hours each day handling their charges, so when a customer wants to buy a hamster, there are no worries about the hamster's jumping out of the owner's hands fearing for his life.

Another striking feature of the pet store staff is its choice of products. They order only what they really believe in. They carry my favorite brand of rabbit and rodent food. Once I asked for a rabbit hutch to use outside, and they found one I liked in a catalog. In no time it arrived at the shop. Many of my rabbits enjoyed spending quality time outdoors in that hutch.

But the most striking feature of the pet store staff is that they make people feel important when they walk in, whether they are buying food or looking to add a new pet to their household.

55. Look in the radiator

I had been asked to do a house call for a new client who owned two ferrets and two cats. When I arrived I asked the owner, Mrs. A., where the ferrets were. She said they were loose in the house and recommended that I check the radiators, as they liked to hide in there. It was summertime so the radiators were off and no danger to the ferrets.

I found a radiator and sure enough, there was a ferret inside. I retrieved her, examined and weighed her, and gave her the necessary vaccination. I returned her to her cage for observation. A small number of ferrets have vaccine reactions and must be watched for several minutes afterward. This is best done in a cage.

We travelled through the large house to find the second ferret and found him in another radiator. After working on him, I placed him in his cage, amused by the thought that this was the first time I ever had to look for my patients in a radiator.

Chapter Six

Fish and Fowl

56. The pond (otherwise known as "Vets can be fish lovers, too.")

As I sat in my backyard, I kept looking at the area where our daughter's playset was, knowing that one day when it was going to be time to get rid of it, I would have a pond in that space. While other homeowners were remodeling their kitchens, I was contacting pond specialists. I found Bob, owner of Unique Aqua Creations. This business has been around since 2001. Bob and his partner, Art, a high school buddy, built my pond.

Bob works as a grocery manager during the day. During the warmer months he services more than 400 ponds in eight counties and has a 90-hour work week. The ponds he builds are lovely, artistic, and show his love for aquatic life.

Bob and Art check the pond monthly when it is warm out and make sure things are running smoothly.

We started with two koi, each 5 inches long, and four goldfish. Now the koi are more than 18 inches long. The goldfish mated, and we soon had 11 of them. They all did well in summer, but winter was a challenge. I had a heater installed that would kick in if the temperature dropped below 38 degrees. I always dreaded the cold weather, as the fish were more susceptible to weather mishaps and pond dysfunctions during that part of the year.

For example, one winter was a blizzard blitz. So much snow fell that it was difficult to simply get to the pond to see if all was well. I tried once and fell into a snow drift, with no one around, and almost froze to death. I finally got up and walked over there and saw that there was no electricity and the pump had stopped running. The pond's surface was partially frozen, and I worried the fish would not survive. Fortunately, they had enough oxygen and free-flowing water, and they all made it! As soon as possible, I had the electricity restored and the pump fixed.

I would count the fish every day. Another year in late fall, I noticed one of my large koi was missing. I finally found her ... in the skimmer! I quickly picked her up and threw her back into the pond. Then I noticed it: she was swimming with an odd, flagella-like movement. She also kept coming up for air. A few days later, she was back in the skimmer. After she had done this over and over, I called and e-mailed fish vets from all over the United States for advice. They recommended everything from putting her in a kiddie pool and taking her to an aquatic vet, to getting a biopsy of the gills, to giving her medicated food.

Bob said she was probably afraid from being attacked by a predator and this was why she was trying to hide in the skimmer. He made a hide box, and she would stick her head in there thinking that she was completely hidden, though she was still mostly visible. He covered the skimmer with mesh, and I ordered a medicated feed to give her for one week. I saw her slowly improve, but as the winter approached, I had my doubts as to how she would do. The weather was growing colder, and I was worried that I would have to stop feeding the fish. Would I have enough time to give her the medicated food so it could help her recover?

Finally, it was spring, and after all of the snow and cold and ice had disappeared, I slowly walked over to the pond. I had never realized how attached I had become to this fish, and as I approached, I hoped she had survived. There she was, swimming with her awkward swagger. I guess in addition to loving dogs, cats, birds, reptiles, amphibians, rabbits, ferrets, and pocket pets, I love fish, too.

57. Freedom versus security

I have many neighbors who let their cats out. Many of these cats come into my yard, gaze at the fish, and catch the baby birds that occasionally fall out of the birdhouses I have scattered in my yard. Then they wander to my back door and look inside, wondering why my cats are imprisoned in the house. My philosophy is that cats should be housed indoors. It is safer for them and the wildlife they would otherwise kill. Not everyone shares this opinion, believing freedom trumps security.

More than once, a neighbor has knocked on my door with an injured baby bird in her hands. "A cat caught it. Could you help it?" A bite from a cat is almost always a death sentence, and though I treated the baby birds, they rarely survived.

Once I found one of my 10-inch goldfish lying dead on the ground beside the pond. I had no idea how it had gotten there and wondered whether a cat, a heron, a raccoon, or a mischievous human was to blame.

I continue to have birdhouses, bird feeders, and a pond with fish. My neighbors continue to let their cats out. It is said that good fences make good neighbors. When it comes to letting cats go out, we are on opposite sides of the fence. In this case, a fence is a small hindrance to a fearsome feline.

58. Old habits die hard.

One of the things my old boss used to say was that parrots live 300 years and they need to be included in wills. Though this may be an exaggeration, they do live longer than dogs or cats: Some may exceed 80 years of age. The parrots that I see as patients range from hatchlings to 45-year-olds. These birds are intelligent and very strong-willed.

When coming over to do a toenail trim on Angie, a 45-year-old Amazon, I needed to be armed with gloves or a towel and ready to place a collar on him so he could be relaxed while I performed my exam. He was one of three parrots who resided in an exotic foliage store surrounded, ironically, by the very plants that would be found in his natural habitat, but he was unable to fly among them.

These birds lived in their cages 100 percent of the time and were intrigued by any outside activities resulting in the clamor of their unified voices. If one could interpret the screeching, it might be that they were yearning for their freedom, to fly through the exotic flowers and to nest in the surrounding trees.

We recently had to do our semi-annual nail trim for these three parrots: Angie, Rocco, 27, and Sadie, 2. Although they lived in separate cages, they loved each other. While clipping Angie's nails, Rocco started screeching at the top of his lungs, sounding just like a siren for the duration of the procedure.

Then, when we trimmed Rocco's nails, Angie started in, sounding even louder and more dramatic. It was a cacophony of parrot voices, deafening to the ear.

Sadie, the sun conure, who was a newcomer to the group, did not get any reaction from the other two while we trimmed her nails. They couldn't have cared less about her. Old habits die hard.

59. My organic block

The block I live on is in love with nature. We have many certified backyard wildlife habitats: chickens, ponds with fish, a maple tree tapped for its syrup, and compost heaps everywhere. We plant native species of plants, do not use pesticides, and place bird feeders and birdhouses in various locations. I even have an owl house in my backyard, along with five bluebird houses. I still have to put up my bat house.

Some of our gardens have sunflowers more than 10 feet tall and milkweed for the butterflies. I am a member of the Backyard Wildlife Habitat Project, which tries to create natural habitats in the backyards of homeowners. These habitats need to have cover for wildlife, places for birds to raise young, a food source, and a water source. My birdhouses are places that many birds covet, from the house wren to the tufted titmouse. The house wren would fill the entire interior of the birdhouse with twigs, then sing at the top of his lungs, hoping to attract a female. When one finally came, she would sigh, "I don't like this location," or, "This is too close to the feeder." The male would work tirelessly day and night, only to be snubbed in the end by his prospective mate.

One neighbor, H., tries to keep her carbon footprint to a minimum by not creating excess waste. She recycles as much as she can, does not use paper towels, and gives all of her table scraps to the backyard hens. She once owned a rooster who would vocalize all day, until a less-evolved neighbor put an end to that.

As a backyard farmer, H. was very practical. She once called on me to look at one of her hens that had been mauled through her cage by a raccoon. The chest contained a large and deep laceration, and a flap of tissue hung from it. This bird was not going to make it, so I suggested I humanely euthanize her. Being a practical farmer, H. said, "No, thanks. Let's just let nature take its course."

Another neighbor also had chickens and had named them all. When her best layer became ill, she was quite distraught, but declined a vet exam. I guess chickens don't seem to have the same power as other pets to get the veterinary help they may need. They are farm animals, and an owner has to ask if it is worth the cost of treatment. For my part, I do not like to see any animal suffering. I even said I would do a low-cost exam just to see if I could help the hen, but I was turned down. Eventually, this hen improved and did well. We think she may have been egg-bound and then passed the egg.

A third chicken owner called me to clip her birds' wings. Though chickens really can't fly well, these were young and had enough lift to get into the neighbor's yard. These four hens were a challenge to catch, as they were loose in the yard. My technician would corner one, and I would try to grab it but was not always successful. Just when I thought I had her, she would get away. This went on for hours, but we managed to catch each one and to clip its wings. Now the owner and the neighbor are happy.

I'm not sure how the hens feel about it.

60. Teflon toxicity

Since birds have air sacs as well as lungs, many chemicals and cooking pans are toxic to them. One of my clients had two parrots—one kept near the window and the other in the living room. The client was up late working on a research paper and had put some milk on the stove for hot chocolate. Absorbed in her work, she forgot about the milk, and it slowly boiled off until the pot was smoking.

The smell carried into her office, and she quickly extinguished the flame, but it was too late for the parrot in the living room, who died shortly after of Teflon toxicity. It had taken only a few minutes to inhale a lethal dose. The other parrot, who had been near an open window, was more fortunate and had enough fresh air, so he had not succumbed to the fumes.

Birds are fragile in one sense, but very strong and mighty in another. They have huge territorial and reproductive instincts. Even tiny finches get picked on savagely by their aggressive cage mates. However, when it comes to Teflon pans and other coated cookware, one should never cook with them near a bird.

Chapter Seven

Medical Leave

61. Life-changing event puts vet practice on hold.

I recently had a life-changing event: I received a kidney from a book group friend. Due to a genetic condition, my kidney function had deteriorated, and I was getting ready to start dialysis.

Suddenly everything changed. My dream of receiving a kidney had materialized. I was stunned and elated, and less than a month later, surgery was performed. I was so touched by this gift of life that I could not put it into words. My donor and I are truly connected by a shared organ. The Bible says the soul resides in the kidney, so I feel we share a common soul.

Both of us were hobbling around for a while, but we improved slowly, until my donor was once again swimming and I was taking longer walks each day. My vet practice had to be put on hold for three months. During that time, I read many books, studied and took on-line vet courses, practiced the saxophone often, and studied French.

The new me was an early bird, up at 4:30 a.m., rarin' to go. I had most of my to-do list finished by 9 a.m., except "practice sax," as I feared I would incur the wrath of my neighbors at that hour.

Taking my early morning walks at 5:45, accompanied by my Pomeranian, George, turned me on to the many beautiful things in my neighborhood that were not noticed during my active work life.

I watched the sunrise while the moon was still in the sky. I looked at the gardens, some very elaborate. I treasured the quiet, as the world had not awakened yet. I listened for the first chirping of the birds and later heard the cicadas as they reached a full crescendo chorus.

Life has no guarantees. Anything can happen, but this experience gave me faith in the good things in life and made the "small stuff" melt away. In no time at all, the three months had gone by and it was back to work, now with a whole new perspective.

62. Will my patients remember me?

So here I was, two months since my surgery and one month left until returning to work. I often wondered what the animals had been doing without me. Did they manage to keep themselves healthy in my absence, or were they taken elsewhere for treatment?

I had many calls from my clients, asking who would come to do a house call during my time off. I started to plan things, such as when to turn my phone message receiver back on and when to start back at the standing clinic. At the same time, I saw how my day was gradually filling up more and more. I practiced the sax longer each day, as my incision was healing and it began to hurt less. I enjoyed transcribing solos, and I resumed my skype lessons with my sax teacher. Whenever possible, I played duets with my mother, a classical pianist, jammed with friends, and met with the sax quartet for rehearsals.

While I was still recuperating, I needed to remind myself to slow down. I was handling too many projects and neglected to rest enough during my recuperation. I was not yet myself, but when the spirit grabbed me, I couldn't turn anyone down.

63. My first day back to work

Starting back on house calls after the three-month absence made me excited and nervous. The outfit I wore was a brand-new teal scrub top with the vet logo and my name sewn onto it. I was also wearing my Vet on Wheels jacket.

My bags were all set up. I had a green bag for general stuff, such as tubes and syringes, gauze and gloves; a blue bag for bandages; an orange bag for fluids; a red bag for blood tests and blood-collection paraphernalia; a purple bag for eye-related exams; and a yellow bag for urine collection. I had a white box for exotics, a smaller one for injectable medications, a cooler for refrigerated things, such as vaccines, and a pink box for oral and topical medications. I also had a blue box for laboratory items, such as slides, culture swabs, and flush. I was so organized ... until I actually got started. Then, eventually, the order decreased. By the end of the day, all of the contents of the boxes and bags had to be reorganized. It stayed very neat, until the end of the next day.

64. Hounds and harriers

Just about a month after my surgery, I began to walk small distances with my kidney donor, Judy, in the South Mountain Reservation, a nature reserve with more than 2,000 acres that is part of the Essex County Park system.

One day, I noticed an ad for a 3-mile race in the fall. The only caveat was that one had to run with a dog. My Pomeranian, George, was 11 years old but still pretty nimble. We started doing the "Couch to 5k" training program.

George was keeping up with me, and I was keeping up with him. I took him for long walks every dawn during my recuperation. This was an ideal time, since the streets were empty and there were no dogs for him to bark at. I had my doubts, however, about doing a race just three months after my surgery.

I filled out the race application and enclosed it in an envelope with a check. I told my husband not to mail it because I was still not sure. The following week, as I was reviewing my checks that had cleared, there it was. It had been mailed after all. I figured it was meant for me to do the race.

As the day approached, I became more apprehensive. Would George be able to run three miles? Would I? How would he act around 150 other dogs? He is not fond of other dogs. Would he instigate a scuffle? I waited until race day to make the final decision: "Let's do it!"

We headed over to the race, battling roadblocks on the way due to other races that were being held in the area. We walked to the staging area to get our goody bag and T-shirt (and bandana for George). We went to the back of the starting line, sure that we would be bringing up the rear.

The race started with no fanfare or loud horn, probably because a loud noise would cause most of the dogs to freak out. We were running at a comfortable pace on this beautiful day; George was slightly ahead of me, and we reached the 1-mile mark. At that time, the elite runners were crossing our path as they approached the finish line. They ran with dogs who were long, sleek, and muscular.

The rest of the race was uneventful, and I noticed George speed up once we rounded the loop and started back toward the finish line. He also dragged me right to the car afterwards. He has a great sense of direction and, apparently, lots of stamina.

George had done well on his first race, and I wasn't so bad myself!

Chapter Eight

Reptiles and Amphibians

65. The iguana lady

Mrs. E. phoned to arrange a house call. She had three enormous, male iguanas. She had to keep them separated or they would fight. One was ailing from dehydration and kidney disease and needed large amounts of subcutaneous fluids weekly. He had been rescued when young, meager in body constitution and suffering from neglect. Ms. E. brought him back to life, and he had grown into a fearsome 16-pound, six-foot-long creature.

Mrs. E. had large cages for all three of the iguanas, and each had toys, branches, and monitors for temperature and humidity that she could remotely check from the living room. Haruki had the whole bedroom to himself, forcing Mrs. E. to sleep on the couch. She was very dedicated to her reptile family and never even took a vacation.

She answered the door, fully covered in leather, including leather pants, leather gloves, and other forms of protective gear. All of her iguanas could bite, and if one did, he could easily amputate a finger. Mrs. E. was no safer than my technician and I were if one of them decided to bare his sharp teeth. She said they were especially prone to aggression when she was menstruating.

Using caution, I examined Haruki and administered the fluids along with an antibiotic injection, with the help of my assistant, Ellie, who happened to be blonde. She was terrified of the patient and hid behind me as I examined him. Then Mrs. E. placed him on a couch, and he would chase Ellie, who kept hiding behind me.

I had brought other technicians, but this iguana seemed to like Ellie. He relaxed and let us administer his treatments, with the television showing "Animal Planet," his favorite show, according to Mrs. E.

Once Mrs. E. visited an animal communicator who told her that Haruki was troubled, but he had a great affection for the blonde woman who came to visit. Now we knew why he was acting that way with Ellie. They had chemistry.

66. Veeck the leopard gecko

One early afternoon I was called to see a leopard gecko at a pet megastore. He had somehow gotten a string around his right hind leg and could not walk on it. I found the lower half of his leg cold and hard, with no blood supply. The string had cut off his circulation, and the leg was beyond saving. The only option was amputation.

I had my technician prepare the site for surgery, and I anesthetized the lizard. Then I removed the lower leg, sutured and bandaged it, and administered antibiotics and pain medicine.

The following week I removed the bandage, and he was healing well, active and eating. Weeks later, he was still there in the cage, up for adoption with no takers. Since I had become attached to this little trouper. I adopted him. My husband named him Veeck, after Bill Veeck, a famous baseball team owner who had lost his leg from wounds sustained during World War II.

Veeck was quick on his feet despite the missing leg. I would let him run around on the floor, and if I became distracted for a second, he was gone, hiding under a bookcase or running out the door. He lived with me for four years, happy and healthy. Then the day came when my transplant nephrologist told me that he had to go. Reptiles carry Salmonella, and I could not take the risk. Sadly, I gave him to a local pet shop, which took him in with open arms. They renamed him Stumpy and were delighted with his positive attitude. Later I learned that he had been adopted by one of my clients who had another leopard gecko I had treated. I know he has gone to a good home. Best of luck, Veeck!

67. The mink (or should I say "stink") frog

On vacation one summer in Maine, we noticed a pond near our hotel. On closer inspection, I saw that there were many frog eggs in clusters floating there. I happened to have a plastic tank with me, just in case I found anything interesting, and I collected some of the eggs and pond water to take back home. Once we were home, I placed them in a larger tank and watched as they eventually hatched into tadpoles and started swimming around.

With time, they grew larger and seemed to be developing well, but the conditions were not ideal, and one did not make it. My daughter was naming the tadpoles and became attached to them, so that when the tadpole died, she cried and said, "He never had a chance to become a frog!"

We buried the tadpole in the backyard and put a little marker over the spot.

The rest of the tadpoles did become frogs, and I looked in my frog atlas to find out what type they were. Looking at their markings and other distinguishing characteristics, I discovered they were the mink variety. These look somewhat like leopard frogs, which are more commonly sold in pet shops.

One day I was cleaning their tank and had to move them to a holding area for a few minutes. I returned them to the cleaned enclosure. Soon after, I noticed a terrible odor in the room and in the entire house. It smelled like a skunk had entered the house and sprayed everywhere. When I researched the problem, I realized that the source of the smell was the frogs, which had become stressed and alarmed by my tampering with them. They had emitted the mink odor, which is a defense mechanism to help them avoid predators. After that, I was very careful when cleaning their tank.

Chapter Nine

The Early Years

68. Get the smelling salts!

When I was in college, I tried to get a part-time job working for a vet. At that time, one needed both small-animal and large-animal experience in order to apply to vet school. I was hired by Dr. A. and looked forward to my first day.

I came to work with high expectations, hoping to learn a lot. Things were going smoothly when suddenly an emergency came in: a German shepherd dog had attacked a pug, and the pug's eye was hanging from the socket. I took one look and almost fainted. They had me lie on an exam table and revived me with smelling salts. I recovered, got up, tended to the dog, and decided that day that I was going to be a vet, in spite of my squeamish response.

I never had a reaction like that again, until I saw a Husky with a bad-smelling tail infection. I lifted the tail, and jumped back ten feet when I saw a mass of maggots nesting under there.

Once I became a vet, things like that were more commonplace, and I grew a thicker skin. Now, almost nothing bothers me.

69. The farm

One of the best experiences I ever had was working on the Jones farm in upstate New York. I needed to have farm experience in order to enroll in vet school, so I applied to various locations, and Mr. Jones hired me. He also hired a male vet student.

My duties consisted of preparing the udders of each of 100 dairy cattle for the milking. After that I would clean the milking machines. There would be a lot of hay to lift and put into the hayloft. We also had to gather the cows from the pasture every morning at the crack of dawn and every evening at dusk.

I wore a bandana around my neck whenever I worked with the cows. I thought it was amazing that each cow knew exactly where to go as she gracefully entered the barn. After the milking, they were allowed to graze in the fields again until the evening milking. We had to yell, "C'mon! C'mon, yah!" and the ladies would slowly rise while chewing their cud and saunter over to the open gate, walking slowly to their stanchions. It was like some parade. I would close my eyes, and all I would see were faces, asses, and udders. Occasionally, a cow would splash me with excrement, another use for my bandana.

Since I was female, I also had to do the dishes and help with the housework, yet my salary was half that of the male vet student's. However, I was glad to work there and loved being outdoors with the cows.

We had no days off as the cows needed to be milked every morning and every evening.

The hay baling followed the morning milking, and that was followed by the evening milking. In between, we ate a big breakfast of pancakes, cooked by Mrs. Jones (who never sat at the table with us and said her husband married her because she resembled a Holstein cow).

After breakfast came the dishes, which I cleaned and put away. Lunch was the big meal, and it was called dinner. The evening meal was smaller and was called supper. We all sat around the table eating ravenously and discussing the day's events.

I always liked this one old cow, whom I named Elsie. She was very bony and very slow. I would gently get her into the barn each day, until one day, she was gone. I asked Mr. Jones, "What happened to that old cow at the back?" and he said that she was now in the freezer. My face fell, but I realized that dairy cows do, indeed, serve us in so many ways, from all of the milk they supply to finally supplying their own bodies to help us sustain ourselves. On a farm, nothing is wasted.

Mr. Jones got his news from the National Enquirer and believed everything Jean Dixon, a psychic and astrologer who predicted JFK's death, wrote. He believed there was a cure for cancer, but that the government was withholding it. If anyone questioned that, he would scream, "I wasn't born yesterday!" and gently kick a cow for emphasis. But Mr. Jones was a genuinely kind man with a love for each of the cows in his dairy barn.

We did have a small break on Sunday afternoons, when we did not have to bale hay. Occasionally I would take the bike out for a ride or go to a movie with the other vet student. I still remember savoring the beautiful mountain views or sitting in the grass just relaxing.

My muscles were never as strong as they were that summer from lifting all of that hay. My health was never better from drinking the milk straight from the bulk tank.

And to think, I never would have had that experience if it hadn't been for the requirement for applying to vet school. Since then, they have dropped that from the list of actions necessary to apply.

These new vet students don't know what they're missing!

70. Vet school and music

Before my first semester in vet school, I was asked to join a band named Kajura. The lead singer, K.J., lived in a house on a hill, near L'Auberge du Couchon Rouge (The Inn of the Red Pig) in Ithaca, New York.

She had a large space for rehearsing. It was sparsely furnished, which let in a lot of light. It also had great acoustics. We played a mixture of jazz-funk-blues-rock originals as well as some well-known tunes.

I was becoming popular among my fellow students, who would come to see me at all of the clubs, as we had many gigs in Ithaca and the surrounding area. One such place was the Rongovian Embassy, a famous club, where we played often.

However, music did not mix well with freshman year studies in vet school, and my schoolwork suffered. I could not memorize origins and insertions of every muscle in the dog's body while practicing for and performing gigs. The other shoe would drop if I did not do something, so, sadly, I dropped out of the band to concentrate on my schoolwork.

Music always was in the background, though, and I soon joined the Cornell Jazz Ensemble and continued to play the sax there. It was less time-consuming and therefore could be sustained without my schoolwork being affected.

The vet school fraternity had a talent show, and I played in it with tunes such as Van Morrison's "Moondance" and Billy Joel's "New York State of Mind."

Recently I visited the Cornell dairy barn during my vet school reunion, and the professor there was giving us a tour of the barn. He saw me and said, "Faith! You played a mean sax back in vet school!"

There was a tinge of regret when I heard that, for I pondered about what I would be like today if I had ventured down that other path instead of the one I had chosen.

The poem "The Road Not Taken" comes to mind. I had considered music as a career but decided to keep it as a hobby instead.

Now, as a busy veterinarian, I am always making time to practice every day, to meet with others to jam or play gigs, and to continue growing and learning. To me, playing the sax is the only time I am truly in flow, where I can immerse myself in the notes and forget what the clock says. It is the connection between myself and the universe, and it helps connect me with others. It stabilizes my mind so I can concentrate on other matters. It is a refreshing breeze, a soothing meditation, a warm embrace, and a loving partner. It helps me be a better person and a better vet.

71. Rough start

When I first graduated from vet school, I worked in an animal hospital that was very mercenary and did not train its new employees well. I was expected to see a certain number of clients per hour, and the more injections I could give, the better. Their ethical practices were not too good, and I did not last there very long.

I left and landed a job in New Jersey. This was also not a great situation.

This boss was a bit old-fashioned, and his wife made the economic decisions, though she was not educated in veterinary matters. That job became a grind, with the staff talking about reincarnation and past-life regression while they ate lunch.

I left there and took another job in New Jersey. This one lasted several years and was when I experienced a professional "growth spurt." I learned for the first time how to talk to clients so that they could really understand me, how to fine-tune my skills, and how to balance work and personal life.

This job had a boss who was a good teacher, a constant joke teller, and also a hard and earnest worker. Then, when I became pregnant and had to be on bed rest due to a high-risk pregnancy, he fired me. Not a great way to end the many years during which I had given my blood, sweat, and tears to the practice.

After I had given birth, I did per-diem work, and then found a full-time job with another employer. My new boss was a workaholic who had a lighter side and was a wonderful mentor. He devoted much of his energy to his practice but was also quite the family man, the skier, and the traveler.

When I first started there, I was the only associate. I had 12-hour days and worked every other Saturday. He eventually relaxed his schedule and hired more vets to work the longer hours so that he was able to take more time off for traveling and hobbies.

I was always making house calls after hours and wondered what it would be like to do them more often. I had worked at the clinic for several years and was there so often that I missed out on much of my daughter's early years.

That was when I decided to devote more time to house calls. I spoke with the boss, and he agreed to let me work part time so I could do the house calls. He was a great sport, giving me many referrals, and I would also send pets to his hospital for work-ups, surgeries, and dentals.

My only question is: What would have happened if I had stayed there full time? There is always *something* to question. I think what I am doing now suits me well. I do not have to be master of everything. Been there, done that.

72. Starting the house call practice and becoming official

The first week I started doing house calls in earnest, things were slow. I walked down my street feeling guilty that I was not at the office, wondering if anyone would call. Eventually, word spread about my service, and the calls started to trickle in. Before too long, my appointment book was filling, and I was looking for technicians. Next, it was time to give the enterprise a name.

While at the clinic one day, I was talking with my dearest work friend Mickey, the bookkeeper. I told her I needed a name for my new house call practice. We bounced around names like Krausman House Calls and Veterinary House Calls 'R' Us, but none sounded quite right. Suddenly I thought, "Well, what am I?" A vet. "What am I doing?" Driving to a house call." I came up with Vet on Wheels. My bookkeeper agreed; it was a great name! That was that.

The next day off, I decided to get my new name protected so no one else could use it in my county. To do this, I drove to the county courthouse. I did not realize until I was about to enter the building that I was carrying contraband in my purse. I always carried a bottle of epinephrine, a bottle of benadryl, and a couple of syringes, in case an animal had a vaccine reaction.

I didn't know what to do. I finally figured I would just explain to the guard if he caught me with it, but I got through security okay.

Next, I had to go into the stacks and search for my proposed business name to make sure it was not already being used. To complete my registration, I needed to get the forms notarized. When I asked about where to do that, the person in charge directed me to the food truck outside the building.

In addition to selling hot dogs and doughnuts, the vendor was also a notary public. For a small fee, he took care of the paperwork. I submitted it, and I was now official!

That day was a memorable one, and I never got caught for carrying those syringes.

73. Dr. Sammy, the master surgeon

When I first graduated from vet school, I felt I needed more surgical experience, so I worked at a low-cost, spay-neuter clinic one day a week. I had a great mentor there, Dr. Sammy, who taught me all of the best methods and techniques. He had a favorite expression, "the dollar dog spay," which referred to the skinny, beagle-type dog who took just a few minutes to spay from start to finish—a dog without any fat or other impediment to a quick and masterful procedure. As the years went by, every time my surgery day would come, I always hoped for "the dollar dog spay."

Dr. Sammy was also big-hearted. He was willing to fix a broken leg on a stray cat for no charge. He was the fastest and most expert surgeon I ever met. For such low prices for a dog and cat spay and neuter, he had to be. I would notice the people driving away in their luxury vehicles, and I would wonder why they had chosen a low-cost spay-neuter clinic. Maybe they knew the great Dr. Sammy was working there. Or maybe they were just cheap.

74. Veterinary economics

There were no courses about economics in vet school. We studied day and night, learned all about animal anatomy and physiology, disease processes, and pathology. We could recite the Merck Veterinary Manual backwards. However, we did not learn about how to work at a job that was profitable and satisfying.

The only thing that would teach us this was a journal called Veterinary Economics. It was complimentary to vet students and was in the cafeteria for the taking. Did I read it? No. I only remember one student who devoured it, reading each article as if it were the great American novel. The rest of us were so removed from the reality of how to make a living and so wrapped up in our studies that we never worried about that sort of thing. We always thought that it would just happen, that we would get dream jobs and make a comfortable salary, and some of us would eventually open our own practices.

Fast-forward 10 years. The economy was in decline. People were watching their spending. Pet care was not on the top of their priority list. Some employers had to cut back on their veterinary staff, decrease the hours of their doctors, and reduce salaries. Even the long-time employees had to make sacrifices.

This pattern at vet clinics was a microcosm of what was happening everywhere else. Whether you were a salesperson selling advertising space or a veterinarian treating animals, it all boiled down to the bottom line. The monthly tallies would come in, and one would see how he or she had done. If an employee did not earn enough money for the practice, he was scolded.

These monthly reports were brought up at doctor meetings, where an employer would say things such as, "We had a terrible month." I understand that it is very expensive to run a veterinary business, and employers were looking out for all of us when they gave us this information, but was I naïve? My thinking was that I had become a veterinarian to treat animals, not be a saleswoman having to perform up to a certain level. The whole idea of 'just caring for the pets and the rest will take care of itself' was a myth.

My current boss did not want to go the way of his predecessors, decreasing hours, salaries, and staff at the animal hospital. Instead, he decided to increase his availability, keeping the office open until 10 p.m. on weekdays, and open on Saturday and Sunday as well. This provided clients with many options, and they were coming in when other hospitals were closed. This enabled him to hold onto his entire staff and even add a doctor. He never gave in to the decline, and he ended up going from being in the red to being in the black.

House calls are my own business, and if things get slow I make sure to send out my reminders, call people who need rechecks, get busy with Chamber of Commerce meetings, and advertise in local papers and online to help market my business. As other house call businesses have entered the arena, competition has become keen, and even the veteran house call vet in my region is noticing a decrease in her appointment schedule. I try to offer more services and improve on client relations. I know it is an opportunity to re-evaluate and restore, to regroup and revitalize, and I am ready for the challenge.

Chapter Ten

Education

75. The effect of illness in pets on the well-being of the elderly

I do many house calls for elderly clients. I began to notice their extreme attachment to their pets. Many had extended families spread out all over the country, but they lived alone for the most part, with only their pet as their constant companion and confidante.

I attended the Ninth International Human Animal Bond Symposium in Rio de Janeiro, where I presented a paper to an international audience of veterinarians, and it was translated into seven languages. This was in September 2001, immediately after 9/11. I had come to Rio on September 8, although the meeting did not start until September 13. Many speakers were unable to attend because their planes were turned around or flights were cancelled. The keynote speaker was unable to come. All in all, it felt surreal being in a foreign country while such a horrible tragedy was occurring back home.

My paper showed that older people, with a smaller social network, were quite reliant on their pets for their sense of well-being. Older individuals would have to get up to take care of their pet, walk the dog, clean the cat's litter box, go to the store for pet food, and would need to get their pet to the veterinarian if the animal became ill.

As part of my research I distributed a questionnaire to two groups. One group consisted of elderly clients and the other a group of younger clients as a control. I asked questions such as, "How often do you socialize with others?" and "Does your family visit often?" and "What do you do when your pet is sick?" My findings were that the elderly respondents were less social, had less contact with family, and were very upset by their pets' illnesses. For some of the elderly, their pet was often the only living thing they interacted with during the course of an entire day.

In my study, I saw that when a pet was ill, the elderly owner felt it, too. In one instance, I saw a dog owned by a 98-year-old woman. He had eaten chocolate and was very sick. I treated him at his home, administering IV fluids and supportive care. I noticed that his owner, a woman who was usually in front of the television watching golf and nursing a highball, was in bed with the lights out. She was so devastated by her dog's condition she was unable to get out of bed. The visiting nurse explained that the owner was beside herself with grief. After I treated the dog and he recovered, the owner did, too, and soon they were both back in front of the television watching golf (but only the owner was sipping the highball).

I demonstrated in my paper that when a pet is ill, the elderly owner was very affected, even becoming ill himself. The control group would have other support systems to help its participants through a rough time and were not affected in this way.

My study inferred that pets have at times become substitutes for human companionship and have to do the work of soul mate, spouse, parent, sibling, child, and friend. This is a sad commentary on our culture, which leaves its elderly isolated with only their pets for comfort.

I once visited the home of an elderly woman with a parakeet whom she loved dearly. There were photographs all over the apartment of her 25 grandchildren. Yet, she was alone in an apartment building with her little parakeet for her social support. This was just one of many house calls I noted that were a sign of the times.

76. Light My Way Career Day

Every year I am asked to talk to a group of young students ranging in age from 5 to 10. It is called Career Day, and many professionals from basketball players, to journalists, to caterers, to scientists come to this special event to show these children that they can become anything they want if they work at it.

I give a speech about my field of veterinary medicine and show the various tools I use to examine a pet. Beforehand, I receive a stack of papers with information on the children. Each child has to fill out a form saying what he or she likes to do and why he or she wants to be a veterinarian. Here are a few examples:

1. What do you love to do?

    - I love butterflies, the park, school, playing dinosaurs.
    - I love to clean my room, clean my bathroom, watch TV, kitchen.
    - Ride my bike, play with toys.

2. Do you know anyone with a job? If so, do they like their work? Do they talk about their work to you?

    - Grandma loves her job. I visited her when I was a baby and she tells me about her job.
    - No.
    - Mommy likes (her) job; don't know what she does.

3. Who would you like to meet on career day? Whose job is interesting to you?

    - Veterinarian

Many have sick parents or come from poor homes with little opportunity for recreation. The school is in a depressed, low socio-economic area, and not many veterinarians want to venture into that region. I have taken along my rabbit, dove, and lizard, and sometimes have borrowed assorted animals from the neighborhood pet store.

My sessions are always the most popular. I hand out stethoscopes and have the children come up to listen to the heartbeat of the rabbit, the hamster, and the bird.

One year when I came to talk to them my dove had laid eggs. So I held one up to show the class.

One child took his stethoscope and held it against the egg, and exclaimed, "I hear the baby bird in there!" This was impossible as my dove did not have a mate and the eggs were not fertilized, but he believed it, so I did not want to burst his bubble. Maybe there would be a virgin birth. Who knows?

Chapter Eleven

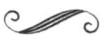

The Shelters and the Rescues

77. The dog rescuers

A wonderful couple in a nearby town was known for rescuing dogs from a county park near their home. Through the years, they had found homes for several dozen dogs and were always finding more that needed rescue.

One day I paid a visit to their house to look at their four dogs. They were *bona fide* mutts, hearty and strong. I loved to see them interact because dogs are pack animals, and it is natural for them to be among other dogs. The older female dog appeared to be calling the shots, and the others deferred to her. They got along quite famously.

When I entered the house, a barking chorus erupted. Then the owner, Mrs. E., would bring each dog to me, one at a time, to examine. At one visit, one of the dogs had a large gash on his neck from an injury he had sustained at the park. I cleaned it up, sutured it closed, and then bandaged it, while he was sedated. He healed well, and in subsequent visits I noted that his hair had grown back and he looked as good as new.

The dogs seemed to have hybrid vigor, a trait that mutts have, enabling them to be stronger and live longer. All of the dogs lived very long, happy, healthy lives. These kind people were the reason.

78. The shelters

Over the years I have occasionally volunteered at local animal shelters. One such facility was set in the woods, surrounded by hills, grass, and trees. Each dog had a name and was listed on a board describing his likes and dislikes, special needs, and warnings if the dog was aggressive. Volunteers would come to walk each dog, who was grateful for any attention. I was asked to examine certain dogs and administer tests and treatments.

One day a Chihuahua needed an eye exam. The staff gingerly removed him from his cage and quickly muzzled him, as he was quite aggressive. I did my exam and prescribed eye medication. I was told that he had been adopted and was going to his new home that day. The next week, I returned, and there he was. When I asked the staff, they said that he was brought back because he tried to bite the child in the house.

Week after week, he would be adopted, then soon returned. Some homes had children while others did not. It made no difference. He would bite anyone. His personality was unchanging, and he couldn't help but be a little terror.

Finally, a staff member who loved Chihuahuas took him home. Some dogs just never realize that if they were just a little friendlier, it might be helpful in getting them a forever home.

There were two cat rooms in the shelter. The cats were everywhere—on windowsills, shelves, the floor, in cat beds, cages, and every nook and cranny. I had to check a diabetic cat by doing a blood glucose level and advise on the correct dose of insulin. The shelter staff was happy to treat this old girl and give her a chance to get adopted. It is hard to be a sick cat in a shelter, among so many other cats. Many needed attention, and the small staff could do only so much.

I found this to be true in a county shelter for which I volunteered. There were 300 cats there and 80 dogs, many of whom were pit bulls. Every Saturday a group of volunteers would come to walk the dogs and socialize them. This helped make them more likely to be adopted.

I think I made a difference volunteering at these places, but, more importantly, seeing those cats and dogs waiting for a home left a big impression on me. Whenever clients ask me where they could adopt a new pet, I always mention these shelters with so many beautiful animals waiting to be loved.

79. The rat rescuer

Rats make good pets because they are clean, smart, and affectionate. If handled gently, a rat will rarely bite. They are very social animals and love to interact with their owners and cuddle or ride on a shoulder. They also love to play. A rat can be trained to respond to its name, use a litter box, climb ropes, fetch, and search for a food item. If a rat escapes from its cage, it will always return.

I have many rat clients, and they provide a home that is fun and enriching. Recently more information has been published about rat nutrition, digestive diseases, dental problems, and obesity. They often get respiratory infections, malocclusion of the incisor teeth, baldness, mammary tumors, kidney disease and pituitary tumors. They are omnivorous, eating both plant and animal foods. They are similar to humans in what they eat, and, like humans, they will overeat due to boredom or stress and become obese.

Ms. E. had several rats. One of her rats, Nymeria, developed a mammary tumor that had to be removed. Later, she had a uterine prolapse and needed to be spayed. Another rat had malocclusion, which caused the incisor teeth to grow abnormally, and she had to have a tooth extracted. Still another rat contracted pneumonia repeatedly, which responded to treatment with antibiotics. Ms. E. is a devoted owner, and on a stormy Sunday afternoon, she attended a lecture on rats I gave at the clinic, listening attentively to my words. If a rat needed rescuing, Ms. E. was ready. She would go to any pet store that had a rat in need, and add the animal to her rat family. When it came to rats and Ms. E, there was always room for one more.

80. The bird (and dog) savior

Sandy is a client who loves birds and rescues them from terrible fates. She would go on craigslist and find dire situations, like the one in which several parakeets and a cockatiel had been placed in a sewer. She quickly rescued them and had me examine all of them.

A test revealed that some were positive for psitticosis, a disease that causes respiratory infections in birds and can spread to humans, so gloves and masks were needed.

The birds were isolated from her "resident flock" and placed in a spare bedroom that was decorated like a beach. There were shells everywhere, as well as beach knick-knacks. I came over weekly to give a doxycycline injection until the treatment was completed several weeks later. They all did well and became part of Sandy's bird family. She had a bird room that housed large aviaries of male parakeets, female parakeets, cockatiels, and parrots.

Sandy did not limit her rescue activities to birds. She also rescued dogs who were usually on their last legs. She would look for the oldest dog up for adoption, regardless of breed or size. She once adopted a 17-year-old Chihuahua who lived another three years, until 20. She loved the Eleventh Hour Rescue because it only dealt with dogs who were old, sick, lame, or had literally one hour to live before being euthanized. Sandy has a heart of gold and a soul linked to these downtrodden animals whom she had to help. There will always be more birds and dogs out there to be saved, and Sandy will be there ready to step in.

Chapter Twelve

My Pets

81. Lemon

I lost my father when I was six. He loved our dog and named him Lemon because he had been adopted from a shelter with worms, distemper, and other problems. He told my mother, "We got a lemon!"

Lemon and I were the same age and very close. He was how I learned about the wonder of having a pet. He could read my emotions. After my father died, Lemon was always there to soothe me. My father had said things like, "Get 'em, boy!" and Lemon would go crazy barking.

He also strictly advised, "Never touch a dog inside of the ears. They don't like that." So, I learned my first canine facts when I was a little girl, with my daddy as teacher.

He trained Lemon to beg, stay, sit, shake hands, and play dead. Lemon was a very good listener and obeyed every command ... until the fateful day when I let him out in the backyard. The gate had been tampered with, was unlocked, and Lemon ran away.

It was a stormy night. He probably just went around the block and was returning when, right in front of the house, a car hit him and sped off. I can still hear the echo of his four cries after he was hit.

Just as she had done eight years earlier, when I had lost my dad, my mom shielded me from seeing him or saying goodbye, telling me the neighbors had taken him to the cemetery.

I suppose that is why I always ask if an owner wants to be present during a euthanasia. The moment is precious, and a goodbye is needed on both sides. It was many years later before I realized Lemon had not really been buried in that cemetery, but I had never asked.

The diary entry on the eve of Lemon's death read, "I love Lemon!" in big letters and red ink.

The next day the entry read, "Lemon is dead!"

82. Herman

My family bought a puppy whom we named Herman. He was a beagle mix, and we got him a day after we lost Lemon. My mother told the man in the pet shop in Brooklyn that she was a widow and her two daughters were devastated by the loss of their beloved pet. The one she wanted was already spoken for, but after hearing her sob story the owner decided she should have the puppy. So Herman was ours.

When Herman turned one, we made him a birthday party. I cooked him a meatloaf cake, and invited two of his doggie pals: George, the beagle, owned by the Tompkin family, and Alfie, the miniature schnauzer, owned by the Napoli family. They played, ran after the ball, and enjoyed the cake. So Herman, George, and Alfie had a grand time at the birthday bash.

We had a family friend come over for a visit when Herman was a bit older, and his name was Herman, too. My mother sternly instructed us not to call the dog by his name, so as not to offend our houseguest. The bell rang, and my mother went to answer it. As soon as she opened the door, the dog jumped on our friend, so she yelled, "Get down, Herman!" The secret was out.

83. The Syrian hamster, or Shmuel's adventure into the depths of music

As a child, I was lucky to be introduced to the Syrian hamster, a breed that was quite popular at the time. My mother's boyfriend, Sam, was a magician and used animals in his act.

One day he came over with one hamster, three white mice, and two ring-necked doves.

Years after my father died, my mother started attending Parents without Partners. There she had met Sam, who was the national vice president of the organization. My mother was a new member, and he held the door open for her as she entered. They had a conversation, and he soon realized he had met his soul mate.

Sam was a magician and used animals in his act, and that is where I come in. I housed his animals and became skilled at caring for them, from hamsters to mice to doves to rabbits.

The mice were named Tom, Dick, and Harry. Tom was a waltzing mouse, who just ran in circles all day. Dick and Harry were type J and K mice, flighty, temperamental, and nippy. I learned all of this by doing research on them.

We named the hamster Shmuel, which is Sam in Hebrew. Shmuel was a character, very animated and lovable. I would let him out all of the time and watch him as he tentatively explored his surroundings.

One day I let him play on our baby grand piano, and he fell into it. There he was, under the piano keys, quite content, but I was petrified that I would not be able to get him out before my mother returned home. I took a carrot and handed it to him to lure him out, but it dropped into the piano. He sat there and cheerfully ate it.

My mother came home and was quite angry when she learned that the hamster was stuck. She called the piano tuner, who did an emergency house call at night, and removed the keys so Shmuel could be freed. He had nibbled on two of the keys, but he was no worse for his escapade.

Sam also gave me a female hamster, Dodee. Shmuel was brown, and Dodee was cream-colored. I learned about sexual reproduction at the age of 10, thanks to my two hamsters.

Every four days the female would come into heat, thereby accepting the male in her domain. He would mate with her for the next few hours, and then he would be removed from the cage. Otherwise she would turn into a devil and attack him. Sixteen days later, she would give birth.

The first time was a disaster. I was not aware that mother hamsters eat their young if they feel threatened, so my hovering over the cage while I watched the birth was not conducive to her feeling safe. I also handled the young, which was a no-no. I watched as she stuffed the seven babies into her cheek pouches and then ate them, one by one. Horrified, I promised to learn from this awful experience and never again to handle the babies or place the mother in an environment that felt threatening.

In a few weeks, she was pregnant again, and this time I did it right. She had 12 young, and they all survived. I kept some of them and gave the rest away to a local pet shop. This kept happening, and I started to acquire a lot of hamsters.

When hamsters reach maturity, they fight if housed together, so I had to get more and more tanks. Eventually, I had 12 hamster enclosures in my room. Each hamster had its own personality. Harry and Archie were brothers and had a bad case of sibling rivalry. Max always ran around the perimeter of my room.

I had a few hamster mishaps, some ending in tragedy. I often placed a hamster in the top drawer of my mother's sewing cabinet and waited for him to climb out and into the bottom drawer so I could say "abra cadabra", and there he was, as if by magic. However, one day it went terribly wrong when I pulled out the drawer too quickly, injuring the little guy. I rushed him to the pet shop, but he died on the way.

My friend wrote a poem:

> *Oh what occurred on August third,*
> *A hamster died today.*
> *It was about two,*
> *We were so blue,*
> *We cried, oh yes,*
> *We cried all day.*
> —Arlene Behar

Another incident occurred on a Saturday morning. I was cleaning the cage of a mother and her young, and I placed them all in the bathroom for exercise. My sister woke up and had to use the bathroom. She slammed the door right on one of the babies, killing him. I was angry with her, but she was not to blame. They were just too easy to get underfoot and into precarious situations.

When I was in the seventh grade, I had enough of them to run an experiment called "Genetics and My Hamsters" for the school science fair.

I mated the brown with the cream, and then back-bred various hamsters. My hypothesis was that the brown hamsters were the dominant color type and that the cream hamsters were the recessive. When I had enough subjects, I did a Punnett Square, which places the genes in a square. In other words, Dd is a brown hamster with a gene for brown and a gene for cream, and dd is cream and DD is brown. I found that the hamsters were never DD, so it must be a lethal combination.

If I mated a dominant (brown) with a recessive (cream), I always got 50 percent brown and 50 percent cream, making the brown a Dd genotype in all cases.

I won first prize in the science fair, and had more than 30 hamsters to show for it. My mother was very tolerant about this, and I was diligent when it came to caring for them, cleaning their cages and giving them my attention. I devised mazes for them with paper towel rollers and had them go into the maze and choose the correct path to the treat at the other end.

I discovered how intelligent these small creatures were. My respect for hamsters has never ebbed, and to this day, I enjoy seeing them at the pet megastores, at the clinic, or on house calls.

As an adult, I bought a hamster, ostensibly for my daughter, but really for me, and I started breeding them again. One day the female got loose in my home office. I put food and water down and saw it had been eaten, so I knew she was nearby. Then I had a great idea: I put the male in the vicinity every day for four days, knowing that hamsters come into heat within that time. Sure enough, on Day Three, when I put him on the floor, the female came out of hiding, unable to resist the strong mating urge that existed within her. I picked her up and put her back into her cage. That adventure was over at last!

The hamsters mated, and many babies were produced. During the female's first litter, she started to stuff the babies into her cheek pouches, and I was painfully reminded of my childhood experience, so we made sure she was comfortable, and eventually she emptied her pouches before any harm could come to the young.

When I had purchased the male hamster for my daughter, he would ride his wheel all night long. Hamsters are nocturnal, meaning they are active in the night and sleep in the day. One should never intrude on a hamster's cage during the day and wake him, as he may become aggressive. If one wants to do this, it must be done with care, paying attention to the hamster's mood. The hamster we had was in my daughter's room and would ride his wheel all night, producing a loud, squeaking sound. My husband could not sleep due to the noise, so he put cooking oil on the wheel to grease the hinges to make it silent. I guess the squeaky wheel really does get the grease!

When I was young I made up poems and songs for each of my pets. One was about Maxwell, my hamster, to the tune of "The Anniversary Waltz."

His cinnamon fur, it gives off a small purr,
And, yet it may seem, that his fur's really cream.
He runs through my room,
and I watch him go zoom,
He finally sits, and he makes a few shits.

> *Then I know that Maxwell is hungry,*
> *and it's time to eat,*
> *It's time for dinner, for dessert it's a treat.*
> *Maxwell will quickly wash his hands and his feet,*
> *And merrily come to din-din.*

Having hamsters when I was growing up made me learn about these small rodents, how they interact with humans and each other, the mating cycle, the gestation period, how they care for their young, how the young mature, and what happens as they age. This education was invaluable to me and has helped me become a vet who truly loves all creatures, great and small.

84. Zack, the rat

I once participated in an experiment for my college class, which was part of the laboratory animal science program. In this experiment, which looked at the effect of zinc deficiency in rats, we had to take white rats and place them into two groups: the control group and the experimental group.

As I looked at the rats, I saw that one stood out and seemed very sweet. He had been placed in the experimental group, so I swapped him out and put him in the control group.

At the end of the six-week period, we had to euthanize the rats and weigh their spleens and livers. Both groups had to be sacrificed, but I took my rat off the chopping block and brought him home. I named him Zack, and he was a great pet. He travelled with me from undergraduate to graduate school.

I could not have Zack in the dormitory, so I handed him over to my boyfriend. Several weeks later, I returned to my dorm to be greeted by a cage with

Zack inside. He was 50 percent lighter and was paralyzed below the waist. I asked my boyfriend about it, and he admitted that he had left him in the woods on his way up to visit me a few weeks earlier. He had left the cage open and hoped for the best. Then he started feeling pangs of guilt, so on his next visit he went back to the drop-off point to see how Zack was doing.

Zack, white and difficult to camouflage, was just sitting in his open cage, an easy target for any predator. He was shivering, frightened, and malnourished. I took him in and hid him from the dorm authorities. When I moved off campus, he came with me.

He was always a good eater, and without the use of his hind legs he grew obese He did well except when the weather was very hot. I would find him in his cage lying on his back to cool off. One day when he was an old man of 5, he died peacefully in his sleep.

85. Raven

During graduate school my roommate had inadvertently let a little black cat follow her home. To get this little fellow to leave, she had put some tuna into a small bowl and placed it outside. He was eating it just as I was coming home. I saw what was going on, and, having begged for a cat and always having heard "No!", I said, "Don't you know the cardinal rule of cats? Once you offer food, you have to take them in."

The kitten came in, was already litter-trained, and very playful. To appease my roommate, I placed a "Lost and Found" ad in the local paper and waited for someone to answer it. Two people came over, but by this time, I was in love. Raven had beautiful eyes, a low meow, a long face, and a graceful stance, hearkening back to his partial Siamese roots. He was *my* cat now. Thankfully, they said he was not the lost pet they were looking for. I never advertised again.

Raven travelled with me from grad school to vet school and from there to Brooklyn, where he stayed while I got situated in my first job. He eventually lived with me as I moved on to other jobs on my rocky, early career path.

He was there during traumatic breakups with boyfriends and difficult situations at work, during big moves and small moves. He was always by my side. I took him with me on a hike to Taughannock Falls in Ithaca, tucked in my backpack.

I once spoke at a Human Animal Bond Symposium, and the speaker before me gave a paper proving that a human companion was not essential to a woman's happiness, as long as she had a cat.

When I met my husband-to-be, Raven accepted him and did not knock books onto him from the bookshelf, which he had done to other suitors. He was with me for many years as the "senior cat," teaching our younger cat, Gin, the ways of the household. He was so much a part of the family that my artistic sister-in-law created a tapestry that read, "We're owned by a cat named Raven."

He eventually developed kidney disease, high blood pressure, and blindness at the age of 20, and he died a year later. I was driving him to the Animal Medical Center to start dialysis when he passed away, just as we were going across the George Washington Bridge, which seemed like the bridge to heaven. It was as if he knew that if I did go forward with dialysis for him, it would have been a tremendous financial strain. So he made the decision for me and left this world quietly and gracefully. I will always have him close to my heart.

86. Patches, the dog with the skin graft

I worked at the ASPCA during the summer of my junior year in vet school. One day there was an "HBT" (hit by truck) that was rushed to the hospital. Her right front leg had a de-gloving injury, which is really what it sounds like.

If one imagines the skin as a glove, her glove came off from the trauma. She also had internal injuries and needed to be stabilized. I became involved in her care, and the doctor in charge decided to make her a teaching case.

There was a big sign on her cage: "DNPTS" (do not put to sleep). Euthanasia was usually the outcome for these unfortunate animals with no one to pay for their medical expenses, but since she was now a teaching case, she received a pass.

We elected to do a skin graft in three steps. First, we took skin from the neck, separated it from the underlying tissue, and connected it to itself. Two weeks later, we walked the proximal portion (closest to the head) over to the top of the right front leg. The third step came two weeks after that. After a circulation bed had formed, we moved the distal portion (farthest from the head) to the bottom of the right front leg. Then we wrapped the skin around the rest of the leg. It took two additional weeks of healing for it to become a normal part of the leg, but she now had the full repair. Since the skin on the neck was furrier than the leg, she looked like she was wearing a leg warmer.

I adopted her, and she was a remarkable dog and very protective and devoted. It was not until she was much older that she developed a brain tumor. After surgery, radiation treatment, and medication, she lived for one more year. Then it was time to say goodbye to my dear friend, but her right front leg had never looked older than when she had first come in on that balmy summer day ... and I have never done a skin graft since.

87. Jaker, the Zum Zum cat

When working at the ASPCA, a cat was brought in with a urinary blockage and was in grave condition. He was dropped off by a waitress at Zum Zum restaurant, a place that had large sausages hanging from the ceiling everywhere. She returned to work and left him for us to treat. He had to be stabilized and immediately unblocked.

The doctor who took care of these emergencies was a genius, an innovator, and one who could think outside the box. He would make his own brand of medication to give greater comfort to his patients. He treated this beautiful Russian blue mix, and then the other veterinarian there started to work on me: "Don't you want this cat? He needs a home. Zum Zum cannot take care of him properly." So Jaker was now mine. He and Raven became great buddies.

I had to place him on a special diet to prevent him from re-blocking, but he did anyway, and eventually needed surgery to cure him. Then he was fine, except for his outrageously big appetite. He would open cabinets to get to his food. He was raised at a place where he probably got to eat sausages all day, and had learned bad habits. He gained too much weight and became very constipated. When he was 17, we considered surgically removing his colon to relieve his condition. But at the same time, he had developed inoperable oral cancer. He did not last long after that. I was grateful for having worked at the ASPCA and crossing paths with such a special cat.

88. The dove saga

Another pet I became acquainted with through Sam's magic acts was the ring-necked dove. He brought over a pair of the birds, and I took care of them.

I saw that the male would do an elaborate display and dance for the female, and both would coo lovingly and regurgitate into each other's mouths as a sign of their true bond.

We saw that they were eager to create a family, and we could not figure out how to accommodate them. Then my sister learned in biology class that one could place a Pyrex dish with grass in it into the cage, so that is what we did. In just a short time, the female began to sit in the dish and lay eggs.

Once the two eggs were laid, a typical clutch size in the dove species, she and the male would share parental duties. They would each spend time sitting in the nest and making sure the eggs were kept warm, occasionally rotating them. When the baby birds hatched and were looking for food, the parents each fed them by regurgitating food into their mouths. It was adorable to watch. These birds were quite compatible, having several clutches through the years.

Sam would take the babies once they were old enough and distribute them to his fellow magicians. The birds were all treated very well. This pair was in it for the long haul, as birds bond for life, and their marriage vows read, "Til death do us part."

Many years later, while working at the clinic, a client brought in a dove with an injured eye. She had seen the bird fly right into the window of a jewelry store, and she had picked it up and brought it in. I examined the bird and treated the injury. The good Samaritan was very grateful and left the bird with me.

Thinking it was a mourning dove, I took it to a rehabilitation center for wild birds once it was healed. The receptionist took one look and said in a gentle voice, "This is a ring-necked dove, not a mourning dove. These doves must be indoors, as they are pets and not wild birds. Good luck with her, and have a nice day." So, embarrassed for not noticing that she did have a ring around her neck distinguishing her from the wild variety, I realized I had a new pet.

We set her up in the house, and I furnished her with a big cage suitable for pigeons, since doves are in the pigeon family. We named her Ring. She became very comfortable in our home and cooed constantly.

Eventually, she started sitting in her food dish, and in a few days, I noticed an egg. A few days later there was a second egg, and she sat on them for several weeks. Then one day she realized, "These are not going to hatch," so she broke them and sat on her perch again. This happened time and time again. I started supplementing her food with calcium to make up for the minerals she was losing when she laid each egg.

Ring was very gentle and sweet, until one day when I brought home another ring-necked dove, which an owner wanted to re-home. I thought they might make a good pair, so I brought them both into the enclosed front porch to let them get to know each other. This was a terrible failure, as I saw her violent side come out. Ring flapped her wings right on the male's body, trying to inflict harm. She turned from a peaceful dove into a bald eagle, aggressive and fearsome. I immediately separated them to protect the male and brought him back to his original owner, apologizing for my bird's bad behavior.

89. Gin and Tonic

When I was working at another animal hospital earlier in my career, two six-month-old kittens came in to be neutered and spayed. They were from a local bakery where they were employed as "mousers." Tonic came in to be neutered, and Gin to be spayed.

After the surgery, Gin became very cold, and my boss had the technicians place a heating element underneath her. Unbeknownst to anyone, the heating unit was malfunctioning, and Gin was too groggy to move off the very hot surface. When it was discovered, she had already suffered burns to her side. The bakery owner elected to give her up, so that we could treat her without charging him.

The cat remained in the hospital and became my project. I had to place her on intravenous fluids, monitor her blood work often, and surgically repair the damage. The blood work showed a dip in her blood cells, including platelets, due to the burn. The surgery to close the open wound on her side was eventually performed, once her condition was stable, and she healed very well. Next thing I knew, she was my new cat. I took her home on April 4th and put her in a bedroom away from Raven, the established cat in the household. I knew that she was negative for feline leukemia virus, but that there was a three-month window during which an exposed cat could turn positive. I could not take the chance of exposing Raven to her. Raven was curious about who was on the other side of the door banging to get out, but he did not seem to mind. On July 4, we retested Gin, and when she was found to be still negative for the virus, we let her out of her room. It was truly Independence Day for her!

90. Deputy

One day at the animal hospital, a four-month-old puppy had been brought in by a good Samaritan. He was very sick and had a high fever. There were two rubber bands around his tail, as if the owner had been trying to dock it. He was black and tan and looked like a mini-Doberman.

The first order of business after he was stabilized was to amputate the tail, since it had been without a blood supply for too long and had become necrotic. Next, he needed to be up to date on his vaccinations and given a new home.

He was fearful and not very friendly. This made adoption a bit difficult. He stayed at the hospital for weeks, and I found myself walking him every day and training him. One day, the boss declared he either go to a home or to the shelter. That was my signal to adopt him. I took him home, and my husband named him Deputy, after Deputy Dog from the cartoon show "Quick Draw McGraw." He would run circles around the other dogs at the dog park and had the grace and speed of a gazelle.

Nervous to have an unpredictable puppy in the house with a toddler, I summoned dog trainers to come to assess him. One said he was too settled and could be dangerous. Another recommended a choke collar and "hanging" him when he misbehaved. I cried on my bookkeeper's shoulder, certain I would have to give him up. Then I consulted a third opinion, an animal behaviorist, who charged $350 to come to my house to look at Deputy. He said he was okay to keep, and that was all I had to hear.

I hired a dog trainer at the beginning and had Deputy learn the rules of the road. He did very well with the trainer present, but as soon as she left, he would lunge at buses, trucks, people, and other pets. I did not make many friends with my neighbors as a result. The trainer said he was "loaded," meaning that he had a lot of unspent energy and a strong herding instinct. He was also very protective of me when he was on a leash. If I took him off of the leash, he would seem to be a different dog, playful and unencumbered by his duty to protect me. It was as if he thought that he was connected to me when he was on a leash and had to guard me with his life.

A more dedicated dog I never owned. If my husband raised his voice to me or tried to embrace me, Deputy would sometimes try to bite him. As the years passed, Deputy continued to mistrust strangers, lunge at moving objects, and chase one of my cats. He would not chase the other one because that cat did not run away. He only responded to cats in motion. Again, the herding instinct would come into play.

He lived a good life. Then one fateful day I was walking Deputy and my other dog, George, and suddenly a dog from across the street broke free from her leash, which was tied to a fence. She leaped right over, like the cow jumping over the moon, and bit Deputy on the neck as George barked frantically. Finally, the owner came out of his house and retrieved his dog.

Deputy was never the same after that. First, he went into shock, and after recovering from that, he lost his appetite and had digestive problems. He became weak and anemic. Diagnostic tests showed no cancer, but an exploratory was performed with an endoscope. His stomach was ulcerated with a possible tumor. I knew it was over, took him home, and euthanized him a day later.

I suspect that the bite had set the wheels in motion. The breed of dog that had bitten him often carries a form of babesia, a blood parasite, and this is transmitted by bites. This may have caused Deputy's demise. I wrote a letter to the owner about not allowing his dog to be unattended while loosely tied to his fence, and I slipped it through his mail slot. Suddenly, I felt a tug on it and heard growling. It was his dog, biting into my letter. I think she may have eaten the evidence.

I will always have a place in my heart for Deputy and think of "Polka Dots and Moonbeams," the tune I played on the sax at a jazz club on the day he died and dedicated to his memory.

91. Dumpy, the White's tree frog

My boss's son was raising White's tree frogs. I love frogs, so I came over to see them. He had hundreds of babies in the tank and was rigging up a screen to prevent them from getting into the filter. I was given four half-inch babies to raise, and I took them home with joy and excitement. I set up a plastic tank as a starter cage. As time went on, I lost one, but three survived.

White's tree frogs are from Australia, New Guinea, and New Zealand. They are so abundant there that they can be found in bathrooms of homes, like one would find a spider in a bathroom in New Jersey.

They are also called dumpy tree frogs because they appear overweight and round like Humpty Dumpty.

The lifespan of a White's tree frog can be up to 20 years. Eventually, all but one frog died. The remaining frog had gone blind, so I had to hand feed him every day. When I went on vacation, I would bring him along, hidden among my suitcases, and smuggle him into the room, placing his travel enclosure in a closet.

All was well, until 4 p.m., when he would start to croak at the top of his lungs, trying to attract a female. I would put a "Do Not Disturb" sign outside the door to avoid having the maid discover the extra guest, and I would spend hours outside our hotel looking for insects for him. I had brought some crickets from home, but they ran out by midweek. Dumpy would always return from vacation renewed and well-fed. And no one ever knew that I had a White's tree frog with me.

92. Frogs

I liked to look for frogs and tadpoles wherever I went. One of my favorite books in grade school was "Frogs and Pollywogs." Growing up, I had a leopard frog as a pet. I made up a song about him to the tune of "Give Him a Great Big Kiss," an oldie by the Shangri-Las:

> *Here comes my frog,*
> *Jumpin' from the chair,*
> *Look how he jumps,*
> *Ooh, so dear,*
> *And every time I see him in the water,*
> *My heart skips a beat goes out of order,*
> *Gonna walk right up to him,*
> *Catch him before he jumps,*
> *Tell him that when I see him,*
> *I get goose bumps.*
> *Tell him that I love him,*
> *Even if he squirms,*
> *I think so much of him,*
> *I'd give him ten mealworms!*

I fed him mealworms that would mature into beetles after going through a pupal stage as fat, white, waxy worms that could hardly move. The beetles would sometimes fly out of the enclosure and take up residence in my house, much to the chagrin of my mother.

Once, the leopard frog escaped. I could not find him, so I put water in several places for him. One day, I was opening a drawer in my dresser and there he was, deceased and just skin and bones. He had his adventure, but he could not survive without water, his life force.

More recently, I became interested in the blue poison dart frog. As I love frogs and I love the color blue, this type of frog is my ideal frog pet. They cannot be touched because their skin emits a chemical that can be toxic.

I went to a reptile show and found a beautiful one and decided to purchase him. He needed a very special habitat, consisting of several layers of substrate, including rocks, dirt, and moss, and air plants such as bromeliads. In addition, the frog would need a special tank with a top that was not aerated too much so that it would stay humid and warm. The frog would need to be fed fruit flies. The breeder had a large container of them, and I bought that along with all of the other accoutrements.

When I returned home, I set up the tank, which took me hours. I fed the frog and watched as his long tongue extended to catch the fruit flies. I noticed that the water-filled clay dish that I had placed in the dirt would eventually be empty as the water somehow was absorbed into the underlying dirt. The humid setup had made the clay bowl permeable to water, and I could not seem to get a bowl that would keep the water from seeping away. Finally, I found a bowl that remained impermeable.

Eventually, I realized that I was running low on fruit flies. I went to several pet shops and found a very poor selection of half-dead flies. I could not believe they would sell such poor-quality food for a frog.

After contacting the supplier of my original fruit flies, I was sent a colony by mail. With this colony, I was to set up fruit fly cultures so I could repopulate my supply. In order to do this, I needed to take 100 flies and put them into another container that had been primed with a yeast template. They would breed, and in a few weeks I would have several hundred.

This procedure was not without accidents, and sometimes a fly (or two or 10) would get out. Then I would have several uninvited guests at the fruit bowl. Finally, I decided to have them send me fruit flies by mail every month. The blue poison dart frog did well, and I thought I would get him a companion. Not realizing that these frogs don't always get along, I went to another reptile show and bought another frog and placed them together.

The new frog was much smaller and, as a result, the larger one began bullying him. The little guy did not do well and later died. It may have been due to stress, the new environment, or an underlying health problem.

I visited the breeder's poison dart frog store in New England and saw many poison dart frogs in various colors, including red, blue, green, and yellow. The different colored frogs were not to breed with other colors, only their own, to keep each color pure and unadulterated.

My poison dart frog was best left as a solitary pet, and he lived for many years in his poison dart frog habitat, happy as a frog could be.

93. Petey

One hot summer day I was asked to see a group of baby peach-fronted conures at a pet megastore. I noticed one of them was cold and being trampled on, while the others had a lot of energy and were bright and alert.

I diagnosed an upper respiratory infection and placed them all on antibiotics. After teaching the staff the proper technique for hand-feeding, I hesitated as I watched the tiny baby bird fall on his side, gasping for air. I made a decision at that moment and implored the manager to give me the baby to treat and monitor to ensure his return to health. He agreed and gave me a tiny bird carrier with a fabric motif of colorful parrots on it, and off I went.

The little bird survived the trip back to the home office, where I set up a cage for him and promptly started medications. He was very weak and needed several tube-feedings a day. I performed many laboratory tests on him, ruling out any infectious diseases.

As the days and weeks went on, he grew stronger and gradually was weaned from the syringe-feedings and was able to eat on his own. As he grew, he became animated and very talkative. By the time he was restored to good health, the pet store bill was so large that the store decided it was more economically feasible to let me keep him. The sad thing is, all of his cage mates did not make it.

We named the bird Petey. He learned how to say, "Petey's a good boy. I love you, Petey," and he made swallowing noises when I took my vitamins. He called

"Deputy!" when I yelled for my dog to come for his walk. He was very attached to me and very lovable, until I took in two wayward Senegal parrots from my boss who had to find a new home for them. As soon as they arrived, Petey went on a hunger strike, would "dive bomb" me when I let him out of his cage, and became aggressive toward me (although he still loved my husband).

All too often emotional problems arise in pet birds, as they are extremely intelligent and frustrated by being in a cage or having to compete with other birds for attention. When we got the Senegals, I moved them to his dining room space, moving him to my home office upstairs.

Petey occasionally started to pick at his chest feathers until he broke skin and induced bleeding. I gently cleaned it and placed a protective collar on him until he healed, and the collar could be removed.

Two years later he was set off by some visitors and voila! He made a 2-inch hole in his chest. This time it required surgical repair and bandaging. Then, two years after that, on the same date, I took him out for a nail trim and noticed he had started feather-picking again. This time I cleaned it, placed the collar back on, and started him on antibiotics, pain medication, and antipsychotic medications to help alleviate his frustration.

He managed to get the collar off and started at it again. After this episode, I put his cage back in its original location in the dining room. Since then I have had to take him to the Animal Medical Center for lupron injections and deslorelin implants to stop the reproductive stress-induced feather picking.

I keep the collar on him when necessary, but take it off when he is more interested in shredding the newspaper then his own feathers. Unfortunately, due to the damage to his pectoral muscles from his picking, he will never be able to fly again. But he is quite the talker, always increasing his vocabulary and always watching every move we make. He even likes to sit and watch TV with us. And he still yells "Deputy" every time I get ready to leave the house. Deputy has been gone for over 5 years.

94. Tyrone

Rabbits have become very popular pets. They are affectionate and can be taught obedience and to use a litter box. They have been selectively bred for coat color and size; many different breeds have resulted, with weights ranging from one to more than 20 pounds.

However, little attention has been paid to selecting for behavior. Unlike the dog, who has become domesticated through centuries of breeding, the rabbit remains just like its wild ancestors. It has fixed action patterns or instincts that have not changed. They are able to use their long ears to hear things humans could never dream of hearing.

As a prey species, they can never relax their guard, even for one second. When a rabbit forages, he must always be ready to flee from an approaching predator. Rabbits' ears may face in different directions to catch all of the sound waves around them. Their eyes are set wide apart, enabling them to see almost 360 degrees around them to be aware of approaching danger behind them.

House rabbits don't need these defenses, but they behave the same way nevertheless. A rabbit sensing danger either freezes or runs like lightning.

I had acquired Tyrone, a 3-month-old checkered giant. He loved to run and hop everywhere. I taught him how to use a litter box and rewarded good behavior with treats, such as romaine lettuce or basil.

Rabbits need plenty of exercise and things to do to keep them happy. Tyrone loved to run up and down the stairs. He would chase my dog, George, whom he mistook for a female rabbit. If a male rabbit spots a potential conquest, he performs a mating dance, circling the female, leaving a 5-foot radius between them. George did not appreciate that too much.

Tyrone would run all over and find new chew toys in the form of cardboard boxes, newspaper, and old books (including an old, treasured book about Mickey Mantle, which my husband did not appreciate). Rabbits sometimes chew on wires and can also ingest foreign objects that could cause an obstruction. It is best to place them in a safe, rabbit-proof room for exercise.

Unfortunately, I had to return Tyrone to the breeder for medical reasons (mine, not his), but I am confident the breeder will take good care of him. He has been raising rabbits for 30 years and is a judge at shows across the country. I know Tyrone may not get the treats, the exercise, or the toys right away, but I hope he either goes to an excellent home or is used for reproductive purposes. I know he'll enjoy that!

95. Ricky

When my daughter was 11, we went to Madison Square Garden for the annual cat show. We had heard that the first floor would have stray cat adoptions. As we looked, we hesitated to make a choice and decided to hold off on that and attend the cat show upstairs.

We passed by several tables of purebred cats. Then we came upon the Burmese cat table. I had some clients with Burmese cats and always thought they were beautiful and smart, with great personalities. I stumbled upon one breeder who said the kittens would be available in a few months. However, we wanted to come home with a new cat that day.

I stopped by the nearby European Burmese table, and there he was. I saw a 5-month-old kitten with a runny nose and tearing eyes, being held by the breeder. The cat was champagne in color with gorgeous stripes of fur across his head. I asked about him and was told he was not for sale as he was sick. So I explained that I was a veterinarian and would bring him back to health. They sold him to us at a reduced cost, and we were thrilled.

Our first stop was to Whole Foods to buy him some roast beef, which he wolfed right down. When we arrived home, he got used to his new digs right away. I treated his upper respiratory infection, and he did very well, gaining weight. He was diagnosed with calici virus, which is a condition affecting the eyes, nose, oral cavity, and respiratory tract. He had very inflamed gums and needed to have all of his incisors extracted before he was a year old. He needed dental cleanings every few years after that.

Ricky has the look and personality of Yoda, strong yet gentle. He will sit on the couch for hours without moving, then when hungry, he will jump up and cry until he is fed. His appetite has led him to be overweight, and we have him on a constant weight-loss program. The biggest challenge is his habit of sneaking over to the other cat's food dish and eating his leftovers.

Ricky is an amazing cat. He is content to eat, drink, sleep, and play. He is like a miniature lion. People say we domesticated the cat so that we can know what it is like to stroke a lion.

He is also a great mouser. If a stray mouse gets into the house, Ricky is on it! He will sit by the spot of the last sighting and just stare until the mouse moves again. Then, he will catch it immediately. He is definitely earning his keep! This is another reason why cats were first domesticated. After all of these generations of breeding, they have retained that basic instinct!

96. Floyd

After I lost my elderly black cat, Raven, everyone would think of me when a stray black cat found its way to the vet clinic. I kept refusing, saying I was not ready, until one day a small, black kitten was brought in, half-drowned in Hurricane Floyd. He was revived, and his owner, a college student, was unable to keep him. So I took him in, naming him Floyd. He was very loving, and he purred loudly as he kneaded my arm. He may have been separated from his mother too young, which made him crave attention. In the beginning, I thought he was deaf from the flood. He never responded when I called him. But one day, I let my cockatiel out, and as soon as she flew to the bookcase, Floyd, who was facing opposite her, turned quickly and began to stalk her. So he apparently got his hearing back.

When Floyd first arrived, my other cat, Gin, was present. She was afraid of the dog, and would run to a high surface to keep safe. Deputy would never chase Floyd though, because he sensed no fear. Floyd would not run away, so what fun was that?

Floyd was very territorial. Once he saw a cat in the front yard and started to growl and hiss. Then he managed to loosen the air conditioner shutters and jump out of a second story window to run after the other cat. I caught up to him and brought him to the clinic for radiographs, blood work, and intravenous fluids. I feared he had ruptured his diaphragm from the fall. He turned out okay and returned home to guard the house. I secured that window, and now he can only yell at the neighborhood cats from inside.

When Floyd grew older, he became very hungry and thin. Blood tests showed that he had hyperthyroidism, a common condition in older cats, resulting in high thyroid hormone levels. He started taking medication for this, and then I considered a radioiodine injection. This would inactivate the tumor, which was benign, and the thyroid levels would normalize. I brought him to Dr. Mark Peterson, "the father of feline hyperthyroidism," for the treatment. He stayed there for four days until he was less radioactive and could be brought home, where he had to be isolated in the basement for three weeks. His litter had to be scooped while wearing gloves and placed in a receptacle away from wildlife. It could not be disposed of for three months. We could only hold him for fifteen minutes a day and not too close to our upper bodies. He was miserable, but after three weeks, he was free.

But he was still thin and hungry, as if nothing changed. Further tests revealed he needed to be treated again, this time with a higher dose. Round two was followed by another three weeks in isolation and another three months of holding onto the litter in a closed receptacle. This time it worked, but a little too well, because due to the treatment he had developed hypothyroidism, which means his thyroid gland was not secreting enough thyroid hormone, and he required daily supplements. But that did the trick, and before long he was back to his old self, eating normally and gaining some weight. All that treatment was certainly worth it.

97. Never bring your 12-year-old daughter with you to a house call at a pet shop unless you are prepared to go home with a new pet.

A new client who owned a small pet shop asked me to examine some puppies. I arrived to find five puppies, some very itchy and missing fur. There were two bichon frises, two white mini-poodles, and one Pomeranian. When my daughter saw the Pom and began to play with him, it was love at first sight.

I examined the puppies and diagnosed mange. This is due to a mite infection that creates dry, flaky skin that is very itchy. It is also very contagious.

I treated the dogs and instructed the owner as to when I needed to come back for the next treatments. At that time, I learned that the owner was going to sell the store, as she was retiring, and it was being converted into another commercial space.

The puppies were allowed to run around in the store, and she was surprised when one of the white poodles turned up pregnant. She was not sure who the father was, but there was a chance it was the other poodle, which was the sibling. The puppies were born and appeared to have trouble walking (a neurological condition called swimmers), and I wondered if this may have been because they were from incestuous parents.

The owner was lacking in some basic knowledge about animal care and maintenance, and I decided to rescue the Pomeranian from this situation. At 6 months old, he had never been outside of the shop. The owner would simply let the dogs run around inside to do their business. This meant he also was not housebroken.

My daughter, who was a Beatles fan, named him George. To be exact, his AKC papers identify him as

George Harrison of Liverpool. George had a lot of training to undergo, but my older dog, Deputy, taught him the ropes, as far as learning not to trust strangers and to bark and growl at them. At first Deputy ignored George, not pleased by this new interloper, but after about four months, it was like a switch was flipped, and he began to play with George and welcome him into the fold.

Years later, George developed a urinary problem. X-rays showed that he had stones in his bladder. He was taken to an interventional radiologist for a percutaneous urolithotomy to remove the stones with a minimally invasive technique. Afterward, he was placed on a special diet to prevent a recurrence. He had to have X-rays every six months for two years, and he remained stone-free.

I think the stones were a result of his deprived beginnings, never having been allowed outside, and having had very little exercise.

George is a wonderful, sweet, 17-pound Pomeranian, afraid of his own shadow and always wanting to sit on a lap. My daughter sure knows how to pick 'em!

98. Real or fake?

Growing up, we always had a yellow canary named Shir (Hebrew for "to sing") who would sing all day, especially when my mother was at the piano. In later years, I always wanted a yellow canary, but never had the opportunity. Then the opportunity arose, in the most surprising turn of events.

Our daughter always loved photography. After a year in Arts and Sciences at NYU, she wanted to transfer to the Tisch School of the Arts, which offered the study of photography. She had to supply a portfolio, and one theme was how to interpret certain statements.

One idea she had was to place real things near fake things. She set up examples, such as a T shirt plus a backpack equal a backpack that looks like a T shirt. Another example was a girl on a bench with her leg sticking out to look as if it were part of the bench.

Finally, an idea she had was to put a yellow canary on the table, photograph it, replace it with a marshmallow, replacing that with a yellow Peep (those marshmallow confections available at holidays). Canary plus marshmallow equals Peep.

I took a trip to the bird store and found a yellow canary. It was a female, which I had wanted for my male at home. I brought her home. Our daughter set up the area by placing a white sheet in the background and a small table in the foreground. She retrieved her camera and lenses, ready for the canary shoot.

Luckily, because the canary had just arrived in our home, she was too stunned to move. I placed her on the tabletop and let go while our daughter took the picture. Right after, I gently picked the canary up and put her into the cage. If I had hesitated even one more second, she would have realized she was free and would have flown away.

The photos came out quite well, and our daughter sent them in. Later, she was informed that she had been accepted at Tisch, and she was ecstatic.

And I was the proud owner of a new yellow canary!

99. To mix metaphors, why buy the cow if the milk is free?

At a pet megastore, I was shown a red factor male canary with an eye injury. These birds are a deep orange in color. After examining him, I found the eye to be permanently damaged and non-visual. I dispensed medication for infection and instructed the staff to apply eye drops. During a follow-up visit, I saw that he was doing well, and was up for adoption. I decided to take him.

They sold him to me for the adoption fee, and I took him home. Only males sing, and I wanted a singer. He was quiet at first, but gradually he began to "perform," first a little, and then all day. He sang whenever he heard music. He sang when he woke up, and before he went to sleep. I thought he would never stop singing.

Then, I acquired the yellow female canary mentioned above. I kept them in separate cages at first and noticed his singing became more desperate and melancholy. He wanted a mate, and there she was, just beyond his reach. I finally housed them together. To my disappointment, the singing stopped. His song was to attract a female. Now that she was there with him, why sing anymore?

Typical marriage.

100. The Senegals or Simon Cowell

One day my boss came in and asked me if I would be interested in adopting his two Senegal parrots. Their loud squawks, their throwing food everywhere, and their feathers' flying finally got to be too much after working an 80-hour work week. I said "Sure," and he brought the cage in holding two beautiful yellow-and-green Senegal parrots.

I had already sexed them and knew the silver-banded one was the female and the green-banded one was the male. My husband helped get the giant cage and the two birds home, and we set them up in our house. At first they were very quiet, but gradually they grew more comfortable and soon were screaming and talking on a daily basis. When they talked, it sounded like someone muttering, "What're ya doin'?'" over and over. When they screeched, it was high-pitched, above the piano's high C. We named them Trixie and Norton, from "The Honeymooners." They are not in love, but rather tolerate each other. No romantic behavior has been observed, and they sit on opposite sides of the large cage. The male seems to like my husband; the female makes kissing sounds as she steps onto my hand. Both are moody and unpredictable, so we always wear hats to protect our ears while they sit on our shoulders.

The cage is next to my music area, and whenever I practice, they eagerly join in. They accompany me whether I am playing alone or with a group, playing jazz or classical, playing clarinet, flute, or sax. They are also my biggest critics. Once I was playing a classical piece, and my mother was accompanying me on piano. They suddenly grew quiet. I told my mom they did not approve of that musical selection, and we tried another one. They became animated and started screaming and singing wildly. I told my mom, "They like that one a lot!"

So I continue to practice, and they continue to give me their opinions. If I post a chorus of a tune on a jazz website, they are always screaming in the background. Their favorite tune, which I play on soprano sax, is "26-2," by John Coltrane. It is the highlight of their day!

Who could have predicted they could be Simon Cowell to my American Idol?

101. The longest-living cockatiel

When I was growing up, my family lived in Brooklyn, and we always rented out the basement apartment.

One of our tenants was Kay. She came with a Doberman and a cockatiel in tow. The Dobie was a show dog, and the cockatiel was very talkative. After becoming acquainted with the bird, we decided to get one for ourselves. We took a trip to the Canary Bird Farm, and found a young male, whom we named Eddie. Eddie would climb on my shoulder, give me a wolf whistle every time I entered the room, and sing, "Shave and a haircut, two bits" incessantly. He was my constant companion while I studied for exams, sometimes driving me to distraction. I tried covering his cage with a blanket to quiet him down, but he continued his discourse undeterred.

Later came Jerry. She was originally purchased for my mom, but my husband and I decided to keep her. She would ride on top of my cat Gin's back like riding a horse and hang out in our front room happily chewing on the wood molding. She would fly over to us to say hello.

After several years, we finally gave her to my mom, and she lived well for a while, being paired with a male and laying eggs at the age of 20. I compared her to Sarah, Abraham's wife in the Old Testament, who became pregnant after the age of 90. That was not to be the case with Jerry, whose eggs were never fertile.

Eventually she became weak, and I took her back and cared for her. She had developed visceral gout and weak bones due to chronic egg-laying and had to be treated with medication. She continued to do well until, at the ripe old age of 26, she quietly passed away. She had a very interesting life and was one of the oldest female cockatiels ever to live.

Epilogue

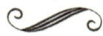

There is nothing like sitting on the couch in Mrs. K's home watching as she gently strokes her 19-year-old dog Sophie, cutting a strand of the dog's hair ever so tenderly, combing the haircoat as if preparing for a dog show. It is such a special moment that I freeze and wish it could last longer, but I have to get up off the couch and interrupt it to perform my exam.

This is something I cannot witness at the office with all of the sights and sounds interfering with the emotional connection that occurs between pet and owner. And that is why I feel that doing house calls gives me a tiny portal into that experience, sharing in the wonder and the mystery of what a pet's love can do for us, and how lucky each of us is to experience it.

As Albert Einstein once said, "The most beautiful thing we can experience is the mysterious. It is the source of all true art and science. He to whom the emotion is a stranger, who can no longer pause to wonder and stand wrapped in awe, is as good as dead—his eyes are closed."

I am glad my eyes are open.